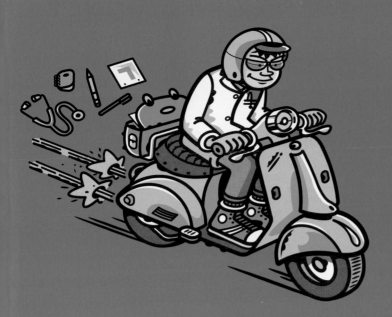

Series editor
Daniel Horton-Szar
BSc (Hons) MBBS (Hons)
GP Registrar
Northgate Medical Practice
Canterbury
Kent

Faculty advisor
Professor Mark Noble
DSc, PhD, MD, FRCP, FESC
Honorary Professor of Cardiovascular
Medicine
University of Aberdeen
Department of Cardiology
Aberdeen Royal Infirmary
Foresterhill
Aberdeen

Cardiovascular System

SECOND EDITION

Toby Fagan
BA (Hons), DPhil
University of Edinburgh
Faculty of Medicine
Medical School
Teviot Place
Edinburgh

First Edition Author
Romeshan Sunthareswaran

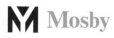 Mosby

London • Edinburgh • New York • Philadelphia • St Louis • Sydney • Toronto 2002

MOSBY
An affiliate of Elsevier Science Limited

Commissioning Editor	**Alex Stibbe**
Project Manager	**Colin Arthur**
Project Development Manager	**Ruth Swan**
Designer	**Andy Chapman**
Illustration Management	**Mick Ruddy**

First edition 1998
Second edition 2002

ISBN 072343249X

British Library Cataloguing in Publication Data
A catalogue record for this book is available from the British Library

Library of Congress Cataloging in Publication Data
A catalog record for this book is available from the Library of Congress

Note
Medical knowledge is constantly changing. As new information becomes available, changes in treatment, procedures, equipment and the use of drugs become necessary. The author, editors and the publishers have taken care to ensure that the information given in this text is accurate and up to date. However, readers are strongly advised to confirm that the information, especially with regard to drug usage, complies with the latest legislation and standards of practice.

Typeset by Kolam, Pondicherry, India
Printed in Spain by Graphycems

The
publisher's
policy is to use
**paper manufactured
from sustainable forests**

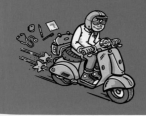

Preface

Recent changes in the way medicine is taught in the UK have meant that much of the responsibility for learning has been given to you, the student. I know I found this difficult to adjust to initially, but it is also liberating—you will have much more time to spend on the areas of medicine that interest you. Cardiovascular medicine is a core subject, and wherever you end up in the medical sphere you will need a good working knowledge of the various pipes, pumps and valves which keep us all going.

I hope that I've managed to make some of the more arcane parts of this plumbing more accessible, and that this book will help you to understand the key concepts. I know that I've learned a lot about the finer points of the cardiovascular system while revising this book, and I hope that you, the reader, will find it an invaluable aid to deciphering lecture notes in the small hours or while struggling with a weighty tome in the library!

Toby Fagan

The Crash Course series aims to provide the essential information in all subjects studied by medical students. The format of the series takes an approach that enhances learning through concise text, comprehension check boxes, and hints and tips boxes.

Every effort was made to ensure that the First Edition presented the latest consensus opinion about the subject. Its success justifies this policy and thus we have tried to make the Second Edition of *Crash Course: Cardiovascular System* even more up to date. Again we hope it will be as comprehensive as possible in relation to the new General Medical Council guidelines for undergraduate medical courses. This is the fundamental reason why Crash Course titles are arranged by body system rather than the previous discipline-based curricula.

In medical schools following the systems-based curricula recommended by the General Medical Council, students will have in-course assessments and examinations on the cardiovascular system. I hope this Second Edition of the *Crash Course: Cardiovascular System* proves to be an even more excellent revision aid than the First Edition, for these examinations.

Mark Noble
Faculty Advisor

In the six years since the First Editions were published, there have been many changes in medicine, and in the way it is taught. These Second Editions have been largely rewritten to take these changes into account, and keep Crash Course up to date for the twenty-first century. New material has been added to include recent research and all pharmacological and disease management information has been updated in line with current best practice. We have listened to

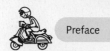

feedback from hundreds of students who have been using Crash Course and have improved the structure and layout of the books accordingly: pathology material has been closely integrated with the relevant basic medical science; there are more multiple-choice questions and the clarity of text and figures is better than ever.

The principles on which we developed the series remain the same, however. Medicine is a huge subject, and the last thing a student needs when exams are looming is to waste time assembling information from different sources, and wading through pages of irrelevant detail. As before, Crash Course brings you all the information you need, in compact, manageable volumes that integrate basic medical science with clinical practice. We still tread the fine line between producing clear, concise text and providing enough detail for those aiming at distinction. The series is still written by medical students with recent exam experience, and checked for accuracy by senior faculty members from across the UK.

I wish you the best of luck in your future careers!

Dr Dan Horton-Szar
Series Editor (Basic Medical Sciences)

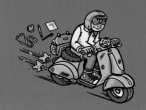

Figure Acknowledgements

Figs 2.16, 2.17 and 2.19 redrawn with permission from WJ Larsen. Human Embryology, 2nd edition. Churchill Livingstone, 1997

Fig. 2.25A redrawn with permission from PL Williams, ed. Gray's Anatomy, 37th edition. Churchill Livingstone, 1989

Fig. 2.25B redrawn with permission from A Davies, AGH Blakeley and C Kidd. Human Physiology. Churchill Livingstone, 2001

Fig. 2.44 redrawn with permission from CP Page, MJ Curtis, MC Sutter, MJA Walker, BB Hoffman, eds. Integrated Pharmacology. Mosby, 1997

Fig. 2.52 redrawn with permission from AC Guyton and JE Hall. Textbook of Medical Physiology, 9th edition. WB Saunders, 1995

Fig. 3.20 redrawn with permission from A Stevens and J Lowe. Human Histology, 2nd edition. Mosby, 1997

Figs 5.22–5.24 and 5.26–5.31 courtesy of T Lissauer and G Clayden. Illustrated Textbook of Paediatrics, 2nd edition. Mosby, 2001

Fig. 5.25 courtesy of T Lissauer and G Clayden. Illustrated Textbook of Paediatrics. Mosby, 1997

Fig. 8.3 redrawn with permission from O Epstein, D Perkin, D de Bono and J Cookson, eds. Clinical Examination, 2nd edition. Mosby International, 1997

Fig. 8.13 redrawn with permission from CD Forbes and WF Jackson. Color Atlas and Text of Clinical Medicine. Mosby Year Book, 1993

Figs 8.16 and 8.17 courtesy of Professor Dame M Turner-Warwick, Dr M Hodson, Professor B Corrin, and Dr I Kerr

Fig. 8.18 courtesy of Professor JJF Belch, Mr PT McCollum, Mr PA Stonebridge and Professor WF Walker

Figs 8.19–28 courtesy of Dr A Timmis and Dr S Brecker

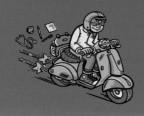

Dedication

By three methods we may learn wisdom: First, by reflection, which is noblest; Second, by imitation, which is easiest; and Third, by experience, which is the bitterest.

Confucius

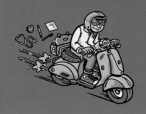

Contents

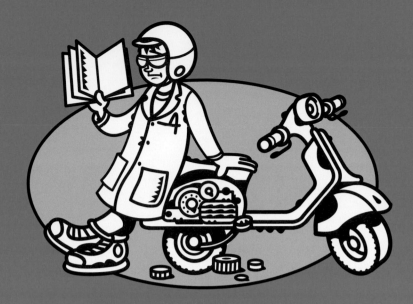

BASIC MEDICAL SCIENCE

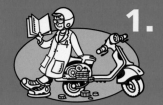

1. Overview of the Cardiovascular System

Why do we need a cardiovascular system?

The cardiovascular system serves to provide rapid transport of nutrients around the body and rapid removal of waste products. In smaller, less complex organisms there is no such system because they can supply their needs by simple diffusion. The human body, however, is too large for simple diffusion to be effective. Evolution of the cardiovascular system provided a means of aiding the diffusion process, allowing the development of larger organisms.

The cardiovascular system allows nutrients:

- To diffuse into the system at their source (e.g. oxygen from the lungs).
- To travel long distances quickly.
- To diffuse into tissues where they are needed (e.g. oxygen to working muscle).

This type of process is called convective transport, and it requires energy. This energy is provided by the heart, with the vessels being the mode of convection.

The functions of the cardiovascular system rely on a medium for transport. This medium is blood, which is made up of cells (mainly red blood cells) and plasma (water, proteins, etc.).

Functions of the cardiovascular system

The main functions of the cardiovascular system are:

- Rapid transport of nutrients (oxygen, amino acids, glucose, fatty acids, water, etc.) and waste products (carbon dioxide, urea, creatinine, etc.).
- Hormonal control, by transporting hormones to their target organs and by secreting its own hormones (e.g. atrial natriuretic peptide).
- Temperature regulation, by controlling heat distribution between the body core and the skin.
- Reproduction, by producing erection of the penis.
- Host defence, transporting immune cells, antigen and other mediators (e.g. antibody).

The heart and circulation

The heart is a double pump. It consists of two muscular pumps (the left and right ventricles). Each pump has its own reservoir (the left and right atrium).

The two pumps each serve a different circulation. A typical blood cell flows first in one circulation and then moves into the other.

The right ventricle is the pump for the pulmonary circulation. Blood is pumped into the lungs, where it acquires oxygen and loses carbon dioxide; it then returns to the left atrium of the heart. This blood then enters the left ventricle.

The left ventricle is the pump for the systemic circulation. Blood is pumped from the left ventricle to the rest of the body. In the tissues of the body, nutrients, and waste products are exchanged. Blood (which now carries less oxygen and more carbon dioxide) returns to the right atrium and then into the right ventricle.

The pulmonary circulation is usually of lower pressure than the systemic circulation as the pulmonary circulation has lower vascular resistance.

The two circulations are operating simultaneously, with blood constantly flowing in each circulation. They can be thought of as being in series, with each circulation supplied by a different pump. This one-way, circular pathway for blood is brought about by the presence of valves in the heart and veins (Fig. 1.1).

The circulatory system is made up of arteries, veins, capillaries, and lymphatic vessels.

- Arteries transport blood from the heart to the body tissues.
- Capillaries are where diffusion of nutrients and waste products take place.
- Veins return blood from the tissues to the heart.
- Lymphatic vessels return to the blood any excess water and nutrients that have diffused out of the capillaries.

The amount of blood ejected from one ventricle during one minute is called the cardiac output. The cardiac output of each ventricle is equal overall, but there may be occasional beat-by-beat variation. The entire cardiac output of the right ventricle passes through the lungs. The cardiac output of the left

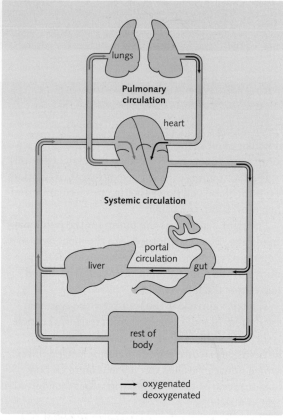

lungs

Pulmonary circulation

heart

Systemic circulation

portal circulation

liver

gut

rest of body

→ oxygenated
→ deoxygenated

Fig. 1.1 Systemic and pulmonary circulations. Unidirectional flow is maintained by valves in the heart, pressure difference in the arterial tree, and valves in the venous system.

ventricle passes into the aorta, and it is distributed to various organs and tissues according to their metabolic requirements or particular functions (e.g. skeletal muscle gets a larger blood supply; the kidney receives 20% of cardiac output so that its excretory function can be maintained). This distribution can be changed to supply demand (e.g. during exercise, the flow to the skeletal muscle is increased considerably).

Blood is driven along the vessels by pressure. This pressure, which is produced by the ejection of blood from the ventricles, is highest in the aorta (about 120 mmHg above atmospheric pressure) and lowest in the great veins (almost atmospheric). It is this pressure difference that moves blood through the arterial tree, through the capillaries, and into the veins. In the veins, the movement of blood is aided by one-way valves.

Arterial blood flow is pulsatile, with a higher pressure during systole than diastole.

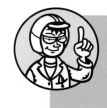 Systole is when the two ventricles contract simultaneously, whereas diastole is when the two ventricles relax together.

- What are the functions of the cardiovascular system?
- How are the two circulations organized?
- How are the flow and distribution of blood through the two circulations governed?

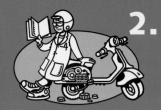

2. Structure and Function of the Heart

Anatomy of the heart and great vessels
Mediastinum

This is the space between the two lungs and pleurae. It contains all the structures of the chest except the lungs and pleurae (Figs 2.1 and 2.2).

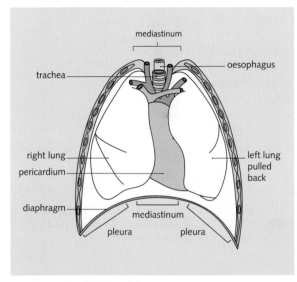

Fig. 2.1 Anterior view of the mediastinum.

The mediastinum extends from the superior thoracic aperture to the diaphragm and from the sternum to the vertebrae. The structures in the mediastinum are surrounded by loose connective tissue, nerves, blood, and lymph vessels. It can accommodate movement and volume changes.

The mediastinum is often subdivided into superior and inferior parts. The superior part contains:

- Anteriorly, the thymus.
- In the middle, the great vessels.
- Posteriorly, oesophagus, trachea, and thoracic duct.

Inferiorly, the mediastinum contains:
- Anteriorly, the thymus.
- In the middle, the heart and pericardium, great arteries, phrenic nerve, and main bronchi.
- Posteriorly, the oesophagus and thoracic aorta.

The heart is in the middle mediastinum, and it has the following relations:
- Superiorly, the great vessels and bronchi.
- Inferiorly, the diaphragm.
- Laterally, the pleurae and lungs.
- Anteriorly, the thymus.
- Posteriorly, the oesophagus.

Fig. 2.2 Lateral view of the mediastinum.

Pericardium

The pericardium is a fibroserous sac, consisting of tough fibrous tissue, enclosing the heart. The outer surface of the heart and the inner surface of pericardium are covered with transparent layers of serous pericardium. Between these layers, there is pericardial fluid.

The base of the pericardium is fused with the central tendon of the diaphragm. The pericardium is also fused with the tunica adventitia of the great vessels entering and leaving the heart. Anteriorly, the pericardium is joined to the sternum by the sternopericardial ligaments.

There are two sinuses (pouches or pockets) in the pericardium; they are formed by the folding of the embryological heart, which produces reflections in the pericardium:

- The transverse pericardial sinus is a recess within the pericardium, posterior to the aorta and pulmonary trunk and anterior to the superior vena cava.
- The oblique pericardial sinus is a blind recess formed by the inferior vena cava and pulmonary veins.

External structure of the heart

The heart lies obliquely about two-thirds to the left and one-third to the right of the median plane (Figs 2.3–2.5). It has the following surfaces:

- The base of the heart is located posteriorly and formed mainly by the left atrium.
- The apex of the heart is formed by the left ventricle and is posterior to the 5th intercostal space.
- The sternocostal surface of the heart is formed mainly by the right ventricle.
- The diaphragmatic surface is formed mainly by the left ventricle and part of the right ventricle.
- The pulmonary surface is mainly formed by the left ventricle.

The heart borders of the anterior surface are as follows:

- Right: right atrium.
- Left: left ventricle and left auricle.
- Inferior: right ventricle mainly and part of left ventricle.
- Superior: right and left auricles.

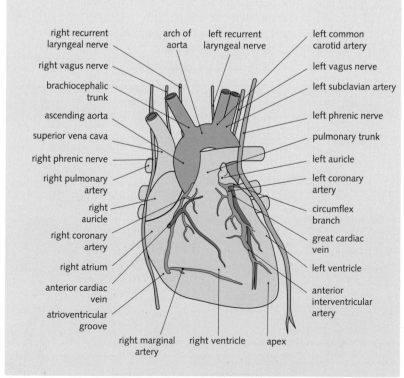

Fig. 2.3 Sternocostal external view of the heart.

right recurrent laryngeal nerve
right vagus nerve
brachiocephalic trunk
ascending aorta
superior vena cava
right phrenic nerve
right pulmonary artery
right auricle
right coronary artery
right atrium
anterior cardiac vein
atrioventricular groove

arch of aorta
left recurrent laryngeal nerve

right marginal artery
right ventricle
apex

left common carotid artery
left vagus nerve
left subclavian artery
left phrenic nerve
pulmonary trunk
left auricle
left coronary artery
circumflex branch
great cardiac vein
left ventricle
anterior interventricular artery

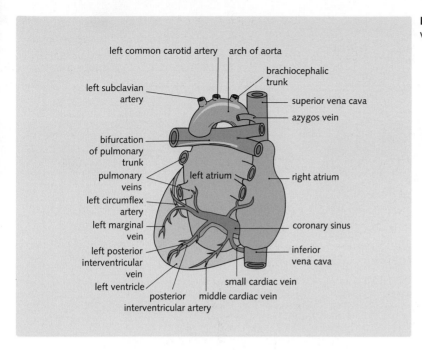

Fig. 2.4 Postero-inferior external view of the heart.

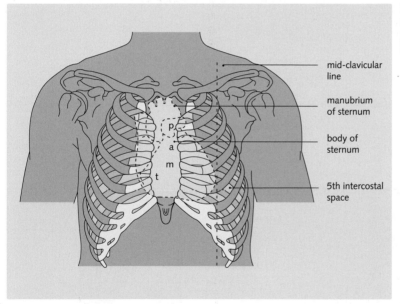

Fig. 2.5 Surface markings of the heart. (a, aortic valve; m, mitral valve; p, pulmonary valve; t, tricuspid valve). See Chapter 7 for auscultatory areas.

Internal structure of the heart

The internal structure of the heart is shown in Fig. 2.6. The right atrium contains the orifices of the superior and inferior venae cavae and coronary sinus.

The right ventricle is separated from the right atrium by the tricuspid (three cusps) valve. The right ventricle is separated from its outflow tract (the pulmonary trunk) by the pulmonary valve. This has three semilunar valve cusps.

The left atrium has the orifices of four pulmonary veins in its posterior wall. The left atrium is separated from the left ventricle by the mitral (two cusps) valve. The left ventricle is separated from its outflow tract (the aorta) by the aortic valve. This also has three semilunar valve cusps.

Coronary arteries

The coronary arteries are shown in Figs 2.7 and 2.8.

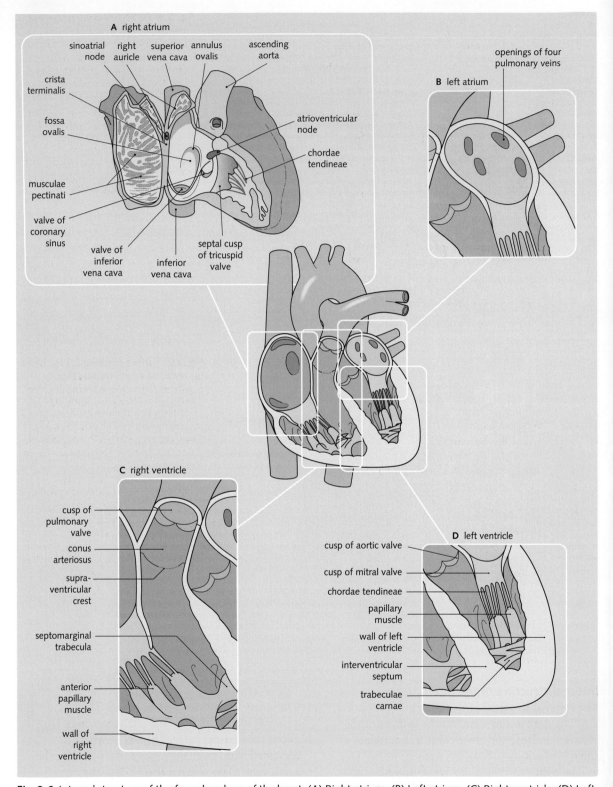

Fig. 2.6 Internal structure of the four chambers of the heart. (A) Right atrium. (B) Left atrium. (C) Right ventricle. (D) Left ventricle.

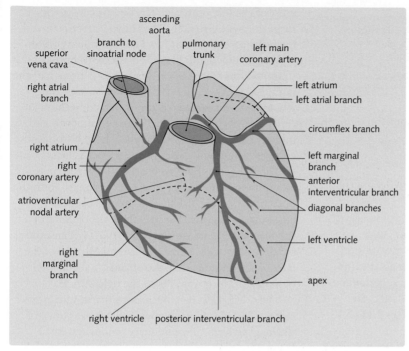

Fig. 2.7 Anterior surface of the heart showing coronary arteries. The left coronary artery has two terminal branches: the anterior interventricular branch (also called the left anterior descending) and the circumflex branch. The anterior interventricular branch supplies both ventricles and the interventricular septum. The circumflex branch supplies the left atrium and the inferior part of the left ventricle. The right coronary artery supplies the sinoatrial (SA) node via the right atrial branch.

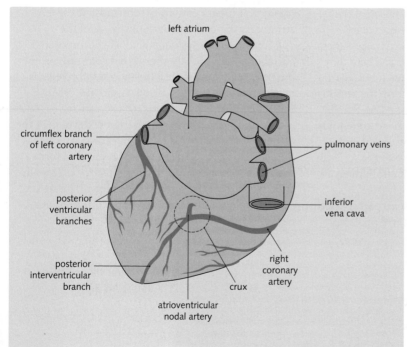

Fig. 2.8 Postero-inferior surface of the heart showing coronary arteries. The right coronary artery gives off a right marginal branch (see Fig. 2.7) and a large posterior interventricular branch. Near the apex, the posterior interventricular branch may anastomose with the anterior interventricular branch of the left coronary artery. The right coronary artery mainly supplies the right atrium, right ventricle, and interventricular septum. It may also supply part of the left atrium and left ventricle. The nodal branch supplies the atrioventricular (AV) node.

The left coronary artery arises from the left anterior cusp of the aortic valve. The right coronary artery arises from the right anterior aortic sinus just above the right anterior cusp of the aortic valve.

Coronary veins

The coronary veins drain mainly into the coronary sinus, which drains directly into the right atrium (Figs 2.9 and 2.10). There are some small veins that drain directly into the heart

Remember that the posterior cusp of the aortic valve has no orifice above it. This is frequently asked about in vivas.

chambers. Generally, these drain into the right side of the heart.

Great vessels

The 'great vessels' is the term used to denote the large arteries and veins that are directly related to the heart. The great arteries include the pulmonary trunk and the aorta (and sometimes its three main branches: the brachiocephalic, the left common carotid, and the left subclavian). The great veins include the pulmonary veins and the superior and inferior venae cavae. The great vessels and their thoracic branches are illustrated in Figs 2.11–2.13.

Development of the heart and great vessels

The heart develops in the cardiogenic region of the mesoderm in week 3. This region is at the cranial end of the embryonic disc. Angioblastic cords (aggregates of endothelial cell precursors) develop and here they coalesce to form two lateral endocardial tubes. During week 4, these tubes fuse together to form the primitive heart tube and the heart begins to pump (Fig. 2.14).

From weeks 5 to 8, the primitive heart tube folds and remodels to form the four-chambered heart. Initially, the primitive heart tube develops a series of expansions separated by shallow sulci (infoldings, Fig. 2.15).

The primitive atrium will give rise to parts of both future atria. The primitive ventricle will make up most of the left ventricle. The bulbus cordis will form the right ventricle. The truncus arteriosus will form the ascending aorta and the pulmonary trunk.

Venous blood initially enters the sinus horns of the sinus venosus from the cardinal veins (a branch of the umbilical vein). Within the next few weeks, the whole systemic venous return is shifted to the right sinus horn through the newly formed superior and inferior venae cavae. The left sinus horn becomes the coronary sinus, which drains the myocardium.

The right sinus horn and part of the venae cavae are incorporated into the growing right atrium to form the posterior wall (Fig. 2.16). This process occurs by intussusception (imagine stretching the opening of a tubular elastic bandage—as the opening widens, the bandage shortens). This gives the smooth wall of the bulk of the atrium, while the original, trabeculated right half of the atrium forms the right auricle.

The original left half of the primitive atrium grows a pulmonary vein, which branches as it moves towards the lungs to form the pulmonary venous system. Eventually, the trunk of the pulmonary vein (which has grown from the primitive atrium) is incorporated (again by intussusception) to form most of the left atrium. As this process continues, more of the pulmonary venous system is gradually incorporated into the atrium. Initially, there is only one orifice, but the process continues until the second bifurcation is reached and four orifices result. Again, the original, trabeculated atrial wall forms the left auricle.

A pair of valves (the venous valves) develop at the orifices of the venae cavae and the coronary sinus. Superior to these orifices, the valves fuse to form a transient septum spurium. The left valve eventually becomes part of the septum secundum. The right valve develops into the valves of the inferior vena cava and the coronary sinus.

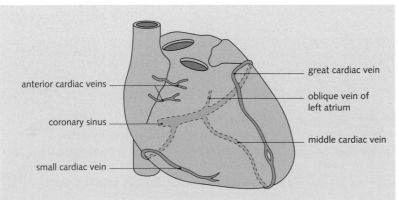

Fig. 2.9 Anterior view of the heart showing coronary veins.

anterior cardiac veins

coronary sinus

small cardiac vein

great cardiac vein

oblique vein of left atrium

middle cardiac vein

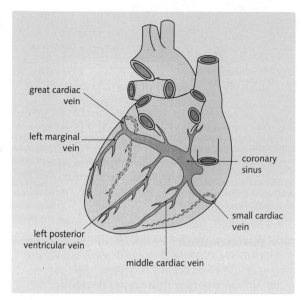

Fig. 2.10 Postero-inferior view of the heart showing coronary veins.

A ridge of tissue, the crista terminalis, forms superior to the right valve marking the edge of the right auricle, and this will eventually form part of the conduction pathway from the sinoatrial node to the atrioventricular node.

In weeks 5–6, the septum primum and the septum secundum grow to separate the right and left atria (Fig. 2.17). These septa are incomplete and leave two openings (foramina or ostia) that allow blood to move between the atria. The septum primum grows downwards from the superior, posterior wall. The foramen (ostium primum) it creates narrows as the septum grows.

The endocardium around the atrioventricular canal (between the atria and the ventricles) grows to form four expansions. These are the left, right, superior, and inferior endocardial cushions.

At the end of week 6, the superior and inferior cushions meet and fuse together to form the septum intermedium, which creates the left and right

Fig. 2.11 The thoracic aorta and its branches.

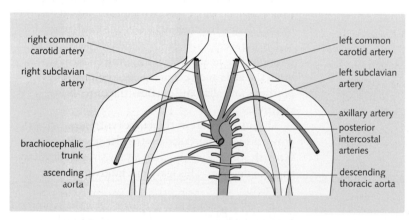

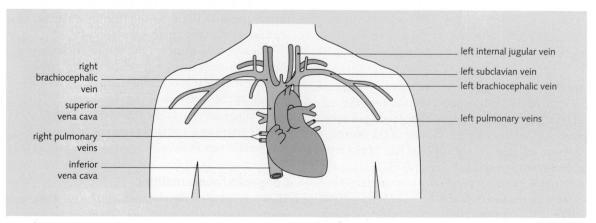

Fig. 2.12 Veins of the thorax.

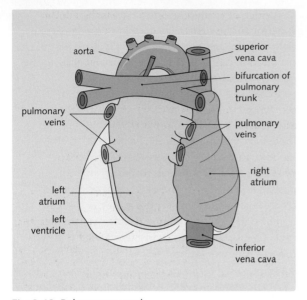

Fig. 2.13 Pulmonary vessels.

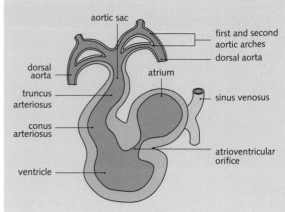

Fig. 2.15 Primitive heart tube as it folds and expands.

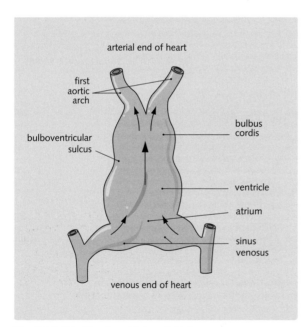

Fig. 2.14 Primitive heart tube at 21 days.

atrioventricular canals (Fig. 2.18). At the same time, the edge of the septum primum fuses with the septum intermedium, closing the ostium primum. However, before complete closure of the ostium primum, cell death in the superior part of the septum primum creates small openings, which join together to form the ostium secundum. This maintains the shunt between the two atria.

While the septum primum is growing, a thicker, septum secundum also starts to form. This septum secundum does not meet the septum intermedium, leaving an opening called the foramen ovale near the floor of the right atrium.

Blood now has to shunt from the right to the left atrium through the two staggered openings in the septum, the foramen ovale and the ostium secundum (Fig. 2.19). At birth, the two septa are fused together to abolish any foramen between the two atria.

During weeks 5–6, the atrioventricular valves develop. The heart undergoes some changes that bring the atria and ventricles into their correct positions and align the outflow tracks with the ventricles.

The inferior part of the bulboventricular sulcus grows into the muscular ventricular septum. Growth stops in week 7 to wait for the left outflow track to develop. This leaves an interventricular foramen.

In weeks 7–8, the truncus arteriosus (the common outflow tract of the heart) is divided in two by a spiral process of central septation, which results in the formation of the aorta and pulmonary trunk. This septum is called the truncoconal septum.

This septum also grows into the ventricles, and it forms the membranous ventricular septum, which joins the muscular ventricular septum. This completes the septation of the ventricles.

Swellings develop at the inferior end of the truncus arteriosus, and these give rise to the semilunar arterial valves.

Congenital abnormalities

The embryological development of the heart is a complex process involving many coordinated steps. Defects arise if the process does not occur correctly.

There are many difficult terms in embryology. Try to understand them by considering what process the term describes. For example, the septum primum is the first (primus means first in Latin) septum to form and septum secundum is the second septum to form.

Congenital cardiovascular abnormalities are the most common congenital defects in live births.

The most common abnormalities include:
- Ventricular septal defect (VSD).
- Atrial septal defect (ASD).
- Atrioventricular septal defect (AVSD).
- Tricuspid and mitral valve defects.
- Persistent truncus arteriosus.
- Transposition of the great arteries (TGA).
- Tetralogy of Fallot.

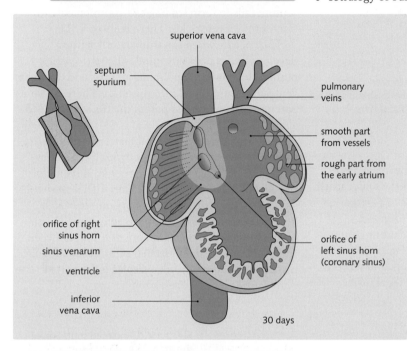

Fig. 2.16 Initial differentiation of the primitive atrium. The primitive atrium derives from two tissues: the rough part from early atrial tissue; the smooth part from venous tissue that spreads as the veins 'push' into the developing atrium. (Redrawn with permission from Larsen, 1997.)

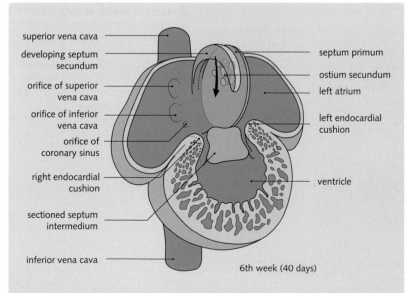

Fig. 2.17 Initial septation of the atria. The septum primum forms at day 33, and eventually leaves a hole (the ostium secundum). The septum secundum develops later at day 40 and is deficient at the foramen ovale. (Redrawn with permission from Larsen, 1997.)

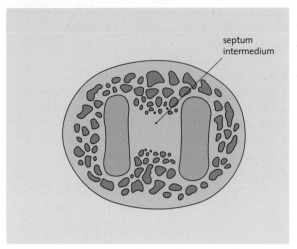

Fig. 2.18 Cross-section of heart at the atrioventricular level. The superior and inferior endocardial cushions fuse to form the septum intermedium. This produces two atrioventricular canals.

VSD can result from failure of the muscular and membranous septa to fuse, failure of the endocardial cushions to fuse (also causes AVSD), or perforation of the muscular septum during development.

There are many types of ASD, including patent foramen ovale and secundum ASD. Patent foramen ovale occurs when the septum primum and septum secundum fail to fuse together at birth, allowing blood to shunt across. A secundum ASD results when the septum secundum fails to grow completely and so does not cover the ostium secundum. When the septum primum and secundum fuse a hole is still present.

AVSD can result from failure of the superior and inferior endocardial cushions to fuse.

Tricuspid and mitral valve defects result from errors in the development of the valves from the ventricular wall.

In persistent truncus arteriosus, the truncoconal septum fails to form leading to a common outflow tract for both ventricles. There is also a VSD.

TGA occurs when the truncoconal septum develops, but it does not spiral. The left ventricle pumps blood into the pulmonary trunk and the right ventricle pumps blood into the aorta. There is also a patent foramen ovale or patent ductus arteriosus to allow blood to mix.

Tetralogy of Fallot is a combination of pulmonary stenosis, right ventricular hypertrophy, overriding aorta, and VSD. The primary problem is failure of the outflow regions to align properly. This causes stenosis around the subpulmonary outlet, which leads to right ventricular hypertrophy. A VSD also occurs because of malalignment, as fusion between the membranous and muscular septum cannot take place. The abnormality also displaces the aorta to the right causing it to be overriding.

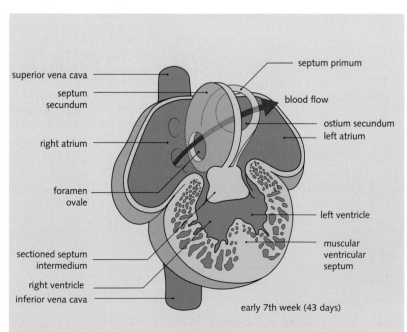

Fig. 2.19 Completed septation of the atria. The septum primum is deficient superiorly at the ostium secundum. The septum secundum is deficient inferiorly at the foramen ovale. Blood shunts from the right atrium through these two holes in the septa to the left atrium. In this way, blood bypasses the lungs in the fetal circulation. As these two openings are staggered, fusion of the septum primum and secundum will abolish any shunt between the atria. (Redrawn with permission from Larsen, 1997.)

These congenital abnormalities are illustrated and further discussed in Chapter 5.

Tissue layers of the heart and pericardium

The heart contains three layers:

- Pericardium.
- Myocardium.
- Endocardium (Fig. 2.20).

Pericardium

The pericardium consists of an outer fibrous pericardial sac, enclosing the whole heart, and an inner double layer of flat mesothelial cells, called the serous pericardium.

The two layers of the serous pericardium are:

- The parietal pericardium, which is attached to the fibrous sac.
- The visceral pericardium (or epicardium), which covers the heart's outer surface.

The serous pericardium produces approximately 50 mL of pericardial fluid, which sits in the pericardial cavity formed by the parietal and visceral layers. This fluid is mainly for lubrication.

The epicardium's thin internal layer of connective tissue contains adipose tissue, nerves, and the coronary arteries and veins.

Myocardium

Myocardium is the thickest layer of the heart, and it consists of cardiac muscle cells. The thickness and cell diameter are greatest in the left ventricle and thinnest in the atria. All the muscle layers attach to the heart skeleton, which provides a base for contraction.

The atrial myocardium secretes atrial natriuretic peptide (ANP) when stretched. This promotes salt and water excretion.

Endocardium

The endocardium has three layers: an outermost connective tissue layer (which contains nerves, veins, and Purkinje fibres), a middle layer of connective tissue, and an inner endothelium of flat endothelial cells.

Heart skeleton

The heart skeleton consists of fibrotendinous (fibrocollagenous) rings of dense connective tissue that encircle the base of the aorta and pulmonary trunk and the atrioventricular openings (Fig. 2.21). The heart valves and cardiac muscle attach to these rings. The heart skeleton forms the base of the heart for contraction.

The skeleton also electrically insulates the atria from the ventricles. The membranous

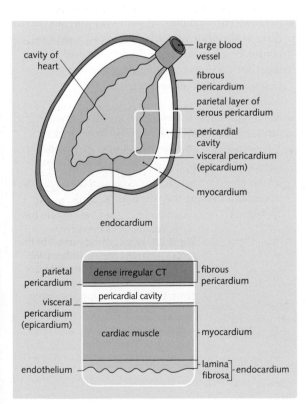

Fig. 2.20 Tissue layers of the heart and pericardium. (CT, connective tissue)

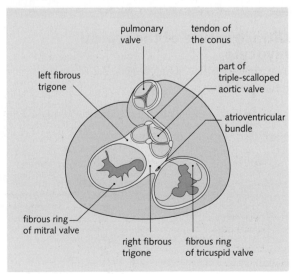

Fig. 2.21 Superior view of the heart skeleton. Vessels and external muscle layers have been removed.

interventricular septum is a downwards extension of the fibrocollagenous tissue, and it contains the bundle of His. The atrioventricular node and the bundle of His form the only conduction pathway through the skeleton and, therefore, the only electrical link between the atria and the ventricles.

Valves

The heart valves are avascular (i.e. they have no blood supply) (Fig. 2.22). This is important if bacteria invade the valves, because there is little immune reaction and infective endocarditis results.

Myocardium
Cardiac myocytes

There are three types of myocytes—work myocytes, nodal cells, and conduction fibres (Fig. 2.23):

- Work myocytes are the main contractile cells.
- Nodal cells generate cardiac electrical impulses.
- Conduction (Purkinje) fibres allow fast conduction of action potentials around the heart (see also p. 18).

The myocardium is innervated by autonomic (sympathetic and parasympathetic) nerves controlled from the brainstem.

Cellular physiology of the heart

Ultrastructure of the typical myocyte

The typical cardiac myocyte (Fig. 2.24) has the following features:

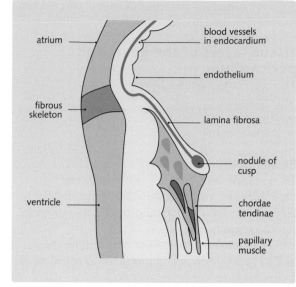

Fig. 2.22 Structure of a heart valve.

- Length of 50–100 μm (shorter than skeletal muscle fibres).
- Diameter of 10–20 μm.
- Single, central nucleus.
- Branched structure.
- Attached to neighbouring cells via intercalated disks at the branch points. These cell junctions consist of desmosomes (which hold the cells together via proteoglycan bridges) and gap junctions (which allow electrical conductivity).
- Many mitochondria arranged in rows between the intracellular myofibrils.
- T (transverse) tubules organized in diads with cisternae of sarcoplasmic reticulum (Fig. 2.25), which enable rapid electrical conduction deep into the cell, activating the whole contractile apparatus.

Fig. 2.23 Types of myocytes. The action potential (AP) is initiated in the nodal cells. It is then rapidly conducted through the Purkinje fibres to the work myocytes where contraction occurs.

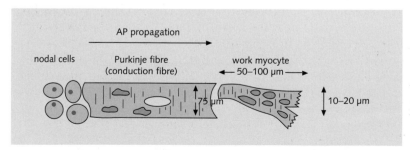

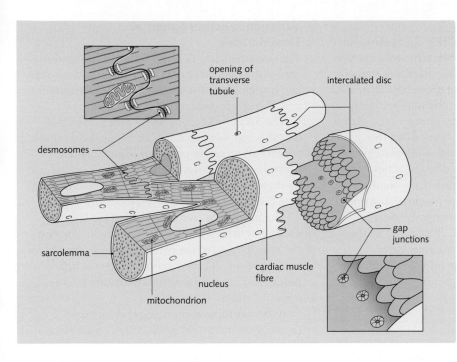

Fig. 2.24 Cardiac myocyte arrangement. Myocytes are branched, and they attach to each other through desmosomes to form muscle fibres. Gap junctions enable rapid electrical conductivity between cells. There is an extensive sarcoplasmic reticulum, which is the internal Ca^{2+} store. The contractile elements within each cell produce characteristic bands and lines. In between each myofibril unit there are rows of mitochondria. Accompanying blood vessels and connective tissue lie alongside each muscle fibre. (Redrawn with permission from Tortora GJ, Grabowski SR. *Principles of Anatomy and Physiology*, 9th edn. New York: John Willey & Sons, 2000.)

- Extensive sarcoplasmic reticulum, which stores Ca^{2+} ions.

Each myocyte contains many myofibril-like units (similar to the myofibrils of skeletal muscle) (Fig. 2.25).

These myofibril-like units are made up of many sarcomeres attached end-to-end and collected into a bundle.

A sarcomere is the basic contractile unit. It is composed of two bands, the A band and the I band, between two Z lines.

The A (anisotropic) band is made up of thick myosin filaments and some interdigitating actin filaments.

The I (isotropic) band is made up of thin actin filaments that do not overlap with myosin filaments. Troponin and tropomyosin are also contained in the thin filaments.

The Z line is a dark-staining structure containing α-actinin protein that provides attachment for the thin filaments.

Excitation and action potentials
Resting membrane potential

The resting membrane potential of a cardiac cell is approximately –80 mV (Fig. 2.26). This value is determined by the distribution of ions across the membrane, and the differential permeability of the membrane. In cardiac myocytes, it is the K^+ gradient that is the major determinant of the resting membrane potential. The potential can be predicted using the Nernst equation:

$$E_K = - 65 \log ([K^+]_{out}/[K^+]_{in})$$

There is a discrepancy between the predicted value and the actual value. This is due to the leakage of small numbers of Na^+ ions inward and K^+ ions outward across the membrane and the action of the enzyme Na^+/K^+ ATPase, which acts to preserve the resting potential.

Digitalis inhibits the sodium pump, partially lowering the transmembrane Na^+ gradient (see Chapter 5).

Action potential

The cardiac action potential (Fig. 2.27) lasts about 300 ms in work myocytes. The arrival of an action potential from a neighbouring cell causes the cell membrane to depolarize and opens Na^+ channels, generating the fast upstroke. This subsequently opens Ca^{2+} channels and this produces the plateau phase. K^+ channels are also opened and this eventually leads to repolarization. The late part of the plateau phase is sustained by the action of the Na^+–Ca^{2+} exchanger. Nerve action potentials, in contrast to the cardiac action potential, last only 3 ms, and they do not have a plateau phase.

The plateau phase (Fig. 2.28), caused by the influx of Ca^{2+}, determines the strength of contraction and it makes the cardiac cell refractory for the duration of the twitch, preventing tetanic contractions.

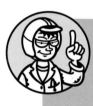

Make sure you can draw a typical cardiac action potential and explain how it is brought about. This is a frequent exam question.

Calcium is the key ion in muscles. Changing its concentration is the basis of most of the actions of the nervous system, hormones, and some drugs that act on the heart and vessels (e.g. noradrenaline from sympathetic nerves increases intracellular Ca^{2+} and increases contraction).

Na^+ channels are blocked by tetrodotoxin, leading to a slower upstroke and action potential.

Ca^{2+} channels are blocked by verapamil, leading to shorter plateau phase and action potential, which weakens contraction. They are opened by adrenaline, enhancing the plateau phase and increasing contraction.

K^+ channels are blocked by caesium, leading to prolonged repolarization.

Variation in action potential
Sinoatrial node

The sinoatrial (SA) node is located in the posterior wall of the right atrium. It is the cardiac pacemaker and is responsible for initiating the depolarization and, therefore, contraction of the whole heart.

The SA node's resting membrane potential is unstable and so when it reaches a threshold value it triggers off an action potential (Fig. 2.29). The upstroke of the action potential is slow because it is mediated by a Ca^{2+} current and not a Na^+ current, as in the fast upstrokes of ventricular myocytes.

The SA node is controlled by the autonomic nervous system. Sympathetic stimulation increases the rate of decay of the resting membrane potential and, therefore, it causes more frequent action potentials. Parasympathetic stimulation has the opposite effect.

A chronotropic agent is one that increases (positive chronotrope) or decreases (negative chronotrope) the heart rate (Fig. 2.30). An inotropic agent is one that increases (positive inotrope) or decreases (negative inotrope) the force of contraction. The action potential varies in different myocytes. Fig. 2.31 shows the action potentials through the conduction pathway.

Excitation–contraction coupling

Contraction of cardiac muscle occurs in a similar manner to that of skeletal muscle.

Active myosins project from the thick filaments (also composed of myosins) and when activated by Ca^{2+} and adenosine triphosphate (ATP), they pull the thin filaments (actin) together to cause shortening. This process involves troponin C and tropomyosin. Full details of this can be found in the title *Crash Course: Musculoskeletal System*.

Contraction is initiated by a rise in cytoplasmic Ca^{2+} as the contractile proteins are dependent upon Ca^{2+} (Fig. 2.32). Relaxation is brought about by a decrease in intracellular Ca^{2+} concentration (written $[Ca^{2+}]$) (Fig. 2.33), and so the duration of contraction is determined by the duration of the plateau. The force of contraction is directly related to $[Ca^{2+}]$ and contractile protein sensitivity to Ca^{2+}. The sensitivity is increased by the initial stretch of the sarcomere (Fig. 2.34).

Hence, the tension/Ca^{2+} curve is displaced to the left by an increased initial sarcomere length (i.e. tension produced during contraction is larger if the fibres are stretched initially; Fig. 2.34). This is the basis for Starling's law (see also p. 27).

Contraction is also dependent on ATP, which is supplied by the mitochondria.

Effect of inotropic agents

Inotropic agents increase force of contractility by affecting cytoplasmic (intracellular) Ca^{2+}. They increase cytoplasmic Ca^{2+} by:

- Increasing Ca^{2+} influx—noradrenaline increases Ca^{2+} entry by opening more Ca^{2+} channels.

- Decreasing Ca^{2+} removal—digitalis inhibits Na^+/K^+ ATPase and, therefore, reduces the Na^+ gradient. This, in turn, reduces the action of the Na^+–Ca^{2+} exchanger. This decreases Ca^{2+} removal from the cell.

Increased heart rate lessens the resting time that the cell has between beats. This also decreases Ca^{2+} removal, causing a gradual increase in cytoplasmic Ca^{2+} and, therefore, force. This is called the staircase or Treppe effect (Fig. 2.35).

The cardiac cycle

Definition

The cardiac cycle (Fig. 2.36) is the sequence of pressure and volume changes that takes place during cardiac activity (Figs 2.37–2.40). A cycle time of 0.9 s is taken at rest.

Events of the cardiac cycle
Ventricular filling (diastole)

The atria and ventricles are all relaxed initially, and there is passive filling of the ventricles. The volume increases until a neutral ventricular volume is reached. Further filling, driven by venous pressure, causes the ventricle to distend. This causes ventricular pressure to rise. Contraction of the atria further increases the filling of the ventricles. However, this accounts for only about 15–20% of ventricular filling at rest. The volume now in the ventricle is termed the end-diastolic volume.

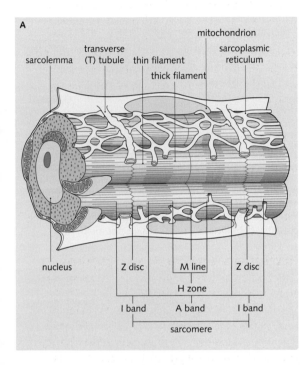

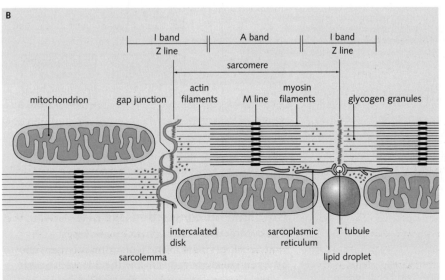

Fig. 2.25
Electronmicrographic appearance of cardiac muscle. (A) Each myocyte has rows of mitochondria in between myofibril-like units. There is also an extensive sarcoplasmic reticulum and T tubule system. (B) Close-up of a myofibril-like unit shows the following bands: A band, myosin with some actin; I band, actin; Z line, attachment point for actin. (Reproduced with permission from [A] Williams, ed, 1989; [B] Davies et al, 2001.)

Ion concentrations			
Ion	Extracellular concentration (mmol/L)	Intracellular concentration (mmol/L)	Equilibrium potential (mV)
Na^+	145	10	70
K^+	4	135	−94
Cl^-	120	30	−36

Fig. 2.26 Intracellular and extracellular ionic concentrations.

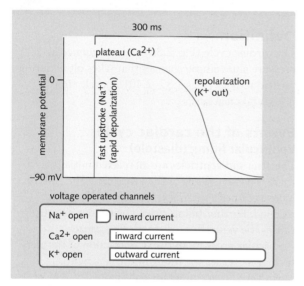

Fig. 2.27 Diagram of cardiac action potential showing the timing of ionic current flow.

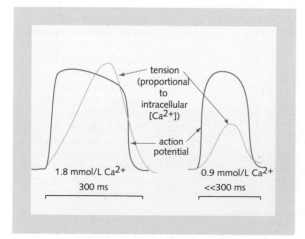

Fig. 2.28 The relationship between cardiac action potential, twitch, and extracellular Ca^{2+} concentration.

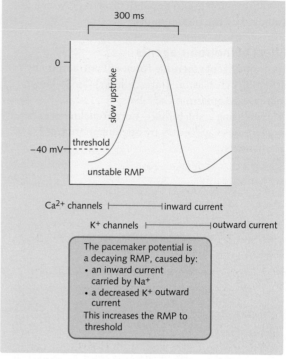

Fig. 2.29 The sinoatrial (SA) node action potential and the generation of the natural pacemaker potential. Voltage-gated calcium channels open once the resting membrane potential (RMP) has decayed above threshold.

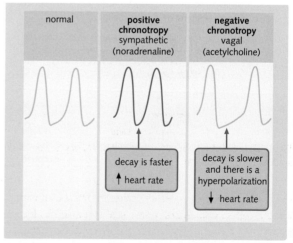

Fig. 2.30 Positive and negative chronotropy. Chronotropes affect the rate at which the heart beats.

Isovolumetric contraction (systole)

The contraction of the ventricles increases ventricular pressure. Ventricular pressure rises above atrial pressure, thereby closing the atrioventricular valves. This creates a closed chamber. As ventricular

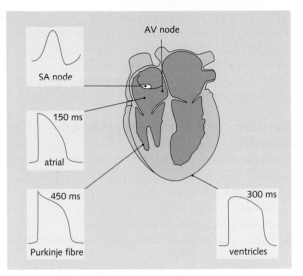

Fig. 2.31 Action potentials in different cardiac myocytes. (SA, sinoatrial.)

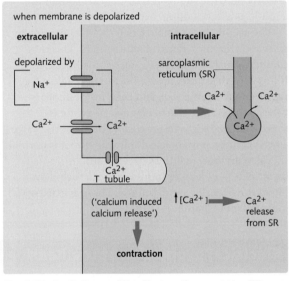

Fig. 2.32 Excitation and its effect on the myocyte. (SR, sarcoplasmic reticulum.)

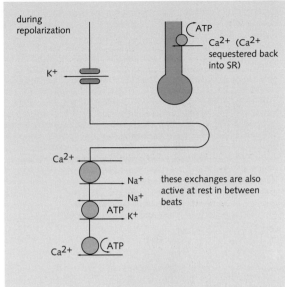

Fig. 2.33 Ion exchanges that take place during relaxation. (SR, sarcoplasmic reticulum.)

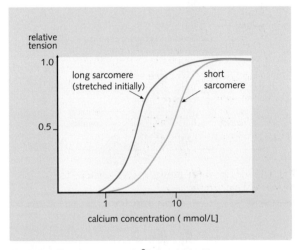

Fig. 2.34 Tension versus Ca^{2+} concentration.

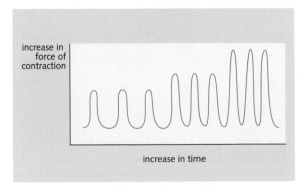

Fig. 2.35 Staircase or Treppe effect. A gradual accumulation of Ca^{2+} within the myocytes leads to an increasing strength of contraction as the heart rate increases.

contraction proceeds, wall tension increases, causing a rapid rise in ventricular pressure. The rate of rise of pressure is a measure of cardiac contractility.

Ejection (systole)

Ventricular pressure rises above arterial pressure, opening the arterial valves. This causes a rapid initial rise in arterial pressure, and then the pressure starts to fall as contraction fades.

The momentum of blood prevents immediate valve closure, even when ventricular pressure falls below arterial pressure. Eventually, the arterial valves

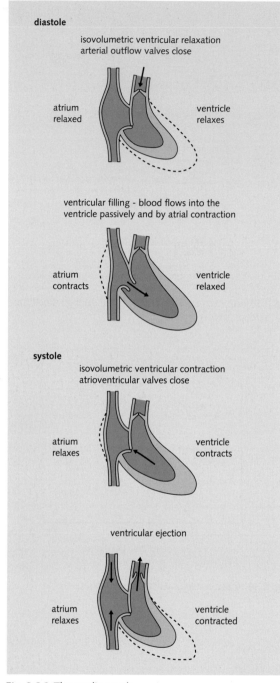

diastole

isovolumetric ventricular relaxation
arterial outflow valves close

atrium
relaxed

ventricle
relaxes

ventricular filling - blood flows into the
ventricle passively and by atrial contraction

atrium
contracts

ventricle
relaxed

systole

isovolumetric ventricular contraction
atrioventricular valves close

atrium
relaxes

ventricle
contracts

ventricular ejection

atrium
relaxes

ventricle
contracted

Fig. 2.36 The cardiac cycle.

close, which creates the brief rise in arterial pressure called the dicrotic wave notch.

The ventricle does not empty completely. There is an end-systolic volume of about 50% of end-diastolic volume, which can be used to increase stroke volume when necessary.

Isovolumetric relaxation (diastole)

The closure of both sets of valves creates an enclosed chamber. The relaxation of sarcomeres plus collagen recoil drops the ventricular pressure. When ventricular pressure falls below atrial pressure, the atrioventricular valves open leading to filling.

Cardiac cycle and normal heart sounds

Four heart sounds can be differentiated (Fig. 2.41):

- First—due to mitral and tricuspid valve closure (the atrioventricular valves).
- Second—due to aortic and pulmonary valve closure (the semilunar/arterial valves).
- Third—due to the sudden rapid flow of blood into the ventricles in diastole.
- Fourth—due to flow of blood into the ventricles due to atrial systole (contraction).

Usually only the first and second heart sounds are audible as a 'lubb–dupp' every beat.

The second heart sound can be split, appearing to be two different distinguishable sounds. This is caused by inspiration increasing right ventricular filling and, therefore, increasing the time taken for right ventricular ejection and delaying pulmonary valve closure. Left ventricular ejection time is shortened leading to faster closure of the aortic valve. This is termed physiological splitting, and it is normal.

Valvular abnormalities (stenosis and incompetence) lead to murmurs, with turbulent blood flow causing extra sounds. These are discussed more fully in Chapter 9.

Electrical properties of the heart

Conduction system

The aim of the conduction system (Figs 2.42 and 2.43) is to allow atrial and ventricular contraction to be coordinated for maximum efficiency.

The steps of depolarization of the heart are as follows:

1. Depolarization is initiated in the SA node (see p. 18).
2. Depolarization spreads through adjacent atrial work cells causing atrial systole in both atria.
3. At the AV node (the beginning of the only electrical pathway through the fibrotendinous ring), the wave of depolarization is delayed by approximately 0.1 s, so that the atria can contract fully.

The cardiac cycle					
	Diastole	Systole			Diastole
Stage	Ventricular filling	Isovolumetric contraction	Ejection		Isovolumetric relaxation
Duration (s)	0.5	0.05	0.3		0.08
AV valves	Open	Closed	Closed		Closed
Arterial valves	Closed	Closed	Open		Closed
Ventricular pressure	Falls then slowly rises	Rapid rise	Rises then slowly falls		Rapid fall
Ventricular volume	Increases	Constant	Decreases		Constant

Fig. 2.37 Summary table of the stages of the cardiac cycle. Changes at fixed volume are referred to as isovolumetric, and precede the later contraction or dilation of the ventricles. (AV, atrioventricular.)

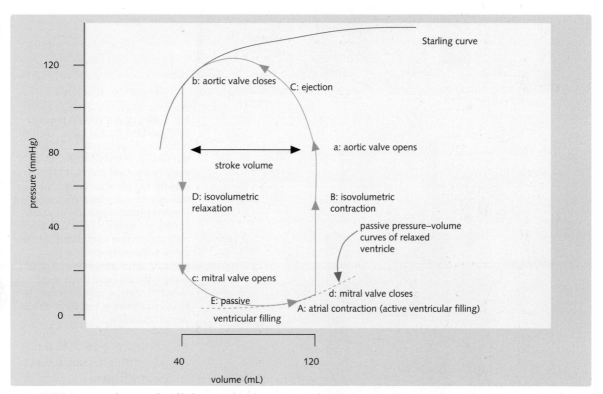

Fig. 2.38 Pressure–volume cycle of left ventricle. The most significant pressure changes occur within the ventricles during the isovolumetric stages.

4. Conduction continues through the bundle of His and its left and right bundle branches. These are very fast conduction pathways.
5. Numerous subendocardial Purkinje fibres distribute the impulse to the work cells in the endocardium.
6. Adjacent work cells then continue the spread to the epicardium to depolarize the whole ventricle.

All cells involved in the conduction process are muscle cells not nerves. They act as an electrical syncytium as they have low resistance electrical connections between them (gap junctions in the intercalated disc).

The SA node controls the heart rate because it has the fastest intrinsic firing rate, but the cells of the AV node and bundle of His can depolarize

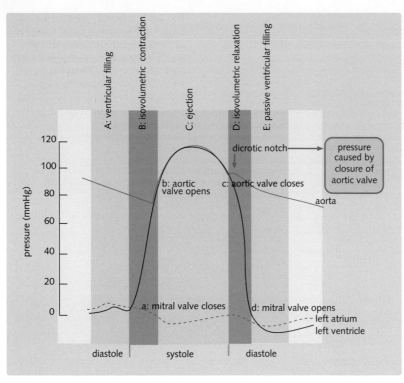

Fig. 2.39 Pressure and outflow in left side of heart. Pressure in the left ventricle increases slightly during left atrial contraction (A). The most rapid increase in pressure occurs during isovolumetric contraction (B). The increase in pressure caused by ventricular contraction closes the mitral valve (a). When left ventricular pressure just exceeds aortic pressure the aortic valve opens (b) leading to ejection (C). Pressure rises to a peak and then falls, leading to aortic valve closure (c). Isovolumetric relaxation then occurs (D) and eventually left ventricular pressure is just below left atrial pressure, leading to the opening of the mitral valve (d). This allows passive filling of the ventricles (E).

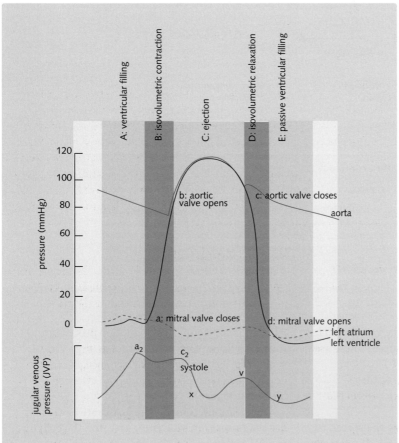

Fig. 2.40 Jugular venous pressure (JVP) and the cardiac cycle. The JVP reflects right atrial pressure due to the close proximity of the central veins to the right atrium and its activity. (a_2, atrial contraction; c_2, movement of the tricuspid valve ring into the atrium when the ventricle contracts—in the jugular vein this may also be due to movement of the carotid artery in systole; v, peak pressure in the atrium due to atrial filling—the tricuspid valve is just about to open; x, x descent due to atrial relaxation; y, y descent due to ventricular filling.)

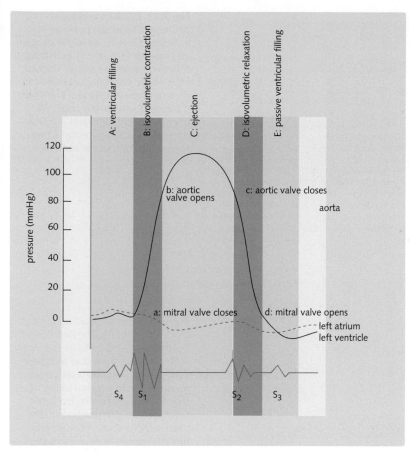

Fig. 2.41 The cardiac cycle and the heart sounds. (S_1, closure of the mitral and tricuspid valves 'lubb'; S_2, closure of the aortic and pulmonary valves 'dupp'; S_3, passive ventricular filling—a low frequency sound; S_4, active ventricular filling due to atrial contraction—a low frequency sound.)

Fibre size diameter and conduction velocity		
Muscle cell (myocyte)	Diameter (mm)	Conduction velocity (m/s)
Atrial work cell	10	1
AV node	3	0.05
Purkinje fibres	75	4
Ventricular work cell	10–20	1

Fig. 2.42 Fibre diameter and conduction velocity of the different cardiac cells.

spontaneously at a slower rate if the SA node ceases to function. Sometimes this occurs in cases of heart block, where the impulse is not conducted properly through the fibrotendinous ring. Ventricular contraction then occurs at an independent rate (about 40 beats/min) to that of atrial contraction.

Heart block is said to occur if there is slow or absent conduction in an area of the myocardium. The action potential can take longer to reach an area of the myocardium and rhythm disturbances can, therefore, result. These are termed arrhythmias.

Re-entry occurs when the wave of depolarization travels back to re-excite an area of muscle that has already contracted (Fig. 2.44). This usually happens as a consequence of ischaemic damage to an area of myocardium. Again this results in an arrhythmia (see Chapter 5).

Electrocardiography

The electical activity of the heart can be measured by performing an electrocardiogram (ECG). This uses electrodes placed on the skin to detect the changing electrical potential within the tissue of the heart.

The characteristic elements of an ECG are:
- P wave—due to atrial depolarization and contraction.
- PR interval—due to conduction through the AV node (approximately 120 ms).
- QRS complex—due to ventricular depolarization (approximately 80 ms).

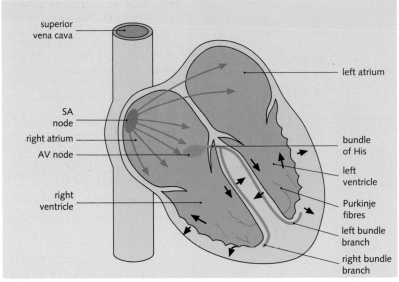

Fig. 2.43 Cardiac conduction pathway. The action potential is initiated in the sinoatrial (SA) node and spreads throughout both atria. It travels through the atrioventricular (AV) node, where it is delayed, and then to the bundle of His. From here it travels down the left and right bundle branches and into Purkinje fibres. The action potential is then spread throughout the ventricles.

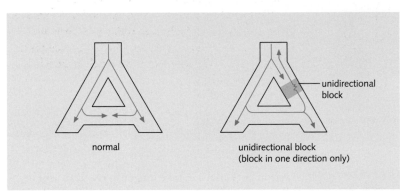

Fig. 2.44 Diagram illustrating heart block and re-entry. The direction of the impulse is indicated by the arrow. A block results from slow or absent conduction. Re-entry results from re-excitation of a region of the heart that has already contracted in the cardiac cycle. It depends upon the presence of a unidirectional block, and it is related to slow conduction and a short refractory period. (Redrawn with permission from Page et al, eds, 1997.)

- QT interval—due to continuing ventricular muscle depolarization (approximately 300 ms).
- T wave—due to ventricular repolarization.

These can be related to the cardiac cycle (Fig. 2.45), and their significance is explained fully in Chapter 8.

Control of cardiac output

Definitions and concepts

Definitions include:

- Cardiac output (CO)—the volume of blood ejected by one ventricle in one minute.
- Stroke volume (SV)—the volume of blood ejected in one ventricular contraction.
- Stroke work (SW)—the amount of external energy expended in one ventricular contraction. SW is the arterial pressure (AP) multiplied by the SV.

Total mechanical work equals the area within the pressure–volume loop. To calculate total energy expended, you must add internal work (i.e. work during isovolumetric contraction), external work (i.e. SW), and heat.

Other definitions are:

- Contractility—the force of contraction for a given fibre length.
- Heart rate (HR)—the number of ventricular contractions in one minute.
- End-diastolic volume (EDV)—the volume of blood in the ventricle just before contraction.
- End-diastolic pressure (EDP)—the pressure of blood in the ventricle just before contraction (preload—see below).
- End-systolic volume—the volume of blood left in the ventricle after contraction.
- Central venous pressure (CVP)—the pressure of blood in the great veins as they enter the right atrium.

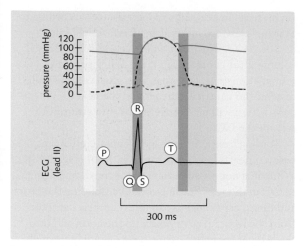

Fig. 2.45 ECG and the cardiac cycle (see Fig. 2.39 for the stages of the cardiac cycle).

- Venous return (VR) —the volume of blood returning to the right heart in one minute.
- Total peripheral resistance (TPR)—the resistance to the flow of blood in the whole system. It is AP divided by the CO.
- Ejection fraction—the proportion of EDV which is ejected by contraction.

The main equations governing CO and work are:

$$CO = SV \times HR$$
$$TPR = AP/CO$$
$$SW = SV \times AP$$

Only three things directly affect CO:
- End-diastolic volume of the right heart (i.e, initial fibre length; this does not apply in pulmonary artery obstruction).
- Resistance to outflow.
- Functional state of the heart–lung unit.

As CO is a product of SV and HR, changes in SV will affect CO. SV is governed by:
- Initial stretch—see Starling's law (see below).
- Contractility.
- AP, which opposes ejection of blood.

But remember that cardiac output is limited by venous return—without integrated regulation of the cardiovascular system, an increased heart rate will be compensated by reduced stroke volume. This also applies in shock.

Starling's law of the heart

'The energy released during contraction depends upon the initial fibre length' (Fig. 2.46). The greater the heart is stretched by filling then the greater the energy released by contraction. This phenomenon is due to the stretch-dependent sensitivity of myocardial contractile proteins to Ca^{2+}, and it is known as Starling's law.

Think of the heart muscle as an elastic band—the more you stretch it initially, the further you can fire it. This will help you understand Starling's law.

Although the initial stretch of the myocardium is produced by the EDV, EDP is easier to measure and the relationship between the two is almost linear. EDP plotted against SV produces the Starling curve (Fig. 2.47). Excessively high filling pressures will cause excessive distension and the relationship is no longer valid. EDP in the right ventricle is closely related to CVP.

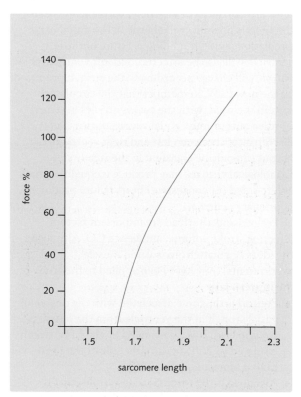

Fig. 2.46 Sarcomere length compared with tension. Increasing the initial sarcomere length increases tension, up to the maximum stretch possible for an individual myocyte.

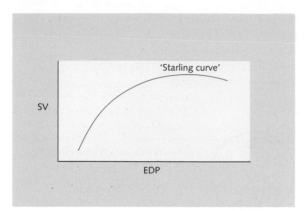

Fig. 2.47 Stroke volume (SV) compared with end- diastolic pressure (EDP). This produces the Starling curve, which shows that an increase in EDP (and therefore end-diastolic volume (EDV) as they have an almost linear relationship) causes an increased SV. There is, however, a limit at which the curve turns downwards and the relationship is no longer valid. The mechanism for this downturn is complex, and it mainly reflects excessive dilatation of the ventricle and valvular regurgitation.

Starling's law matches right and left ventricular stroke volumes. If HR and myocardial contractility are constant, CVP will determine the CO. Although CVP affects the right ventricle, within a few beats the venous pressure will change in the pulmonary circulation and so the filling pressure of the left ventricle will also be affected, and left ventricular output will change according to the stretch produced by the new EDV. Remember that the circulatory system is closed, with the two ventricles in series. Cardiac output must equal venous return, and discrepancies between left and right ventricular output can only be transient in the steady state. Pathological changes may produce inequalities, such as left-sided (or congestive) heart failure producing pulmonary oedema.

Preload and afterload are important factors affecting stroke volume, and hence CO. Although the ideas originate from isolated muscle experiments, they have been applied to the study of the heart *in vivo*:

- Preload is the force associated with the degree of initial stretch in the ventricle from the initial volume load. It is determined by the EDV, which is related to EDP. In the right side of the heart, EDP is almost equal to CVP.
- Afterload is the force (load in systole) that is determined by AP (which is related to the resistance to outflow (i.e. TPR)) and ventricular volume by the Laplace relationship.

An increase in preload will increase CO according to Starling's law. An increase in afterload will initially decrease CO. The heart will have a greater residual volume after contraction. If the filling pressure remains constant, the greater residual volume will distend the ventricle further and the next contraction will be stronger. This is an attempt to restore the CO.

Starling's experiments were conducted on an isolated heart–lung preparation in 1914 (Fig. 2.48). While it is not possible to monitor the determinants of CO in the way Starling could by isolating the heart and lungs, cardiologists can insert a single catheter from the femoral artery back up the aorta and into the left ventricle by passing it retrogradely through the aortic valve. The catheter contains conductance sensors to measure left ventricular volume and a pressure sensor at the tip. This freely records the pressure–volume loops (Fig. 2.49).

Starling's findings in the controlled situation of the isolated heart–lung preparation are important in enabling clinicians to understand the importance of:

- Adequate, but not excessive, filling of the ventricles (e.g. in heart failure, high EDV may be pathological).
- Keeping peripheral resistance as low as possible to maximize CO.
- Maintaining a sufficient level of contractility to maintain life when the previous determinants have been optimized.

When the blood supply through the coronary arteries is compromised, it is important to keep certain methods of increasing CO (especially increased contractility) to a minimum because they increase oxygen consumption of the heart muscle, and, therefore, increase the demand for blood supply and the intensity of ischaemia.

 Starling's law reflects the in-built properties of the myocytes. Remember, however, that the force of contraction can also be affected by other extrinsic factors, e.g. sympathetic stimulation. Starling's law is not the only factor that affects SV.

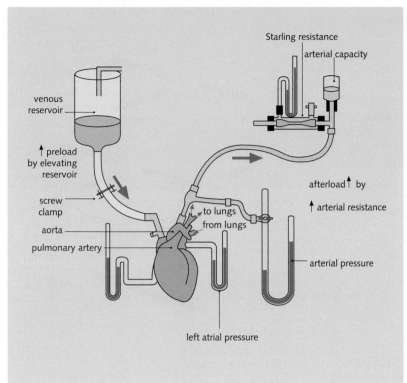

Fig. 2.48 Starling heart–lung preparation. He used an isolated heart–lung preparation and looked at the result of varying end-diastolic volume (EDV) and arterial resistance. EDV is sometimes called preload; arterial resistance is sometimes termed afterload. These terms were not used by Starling in his experiments, but they are sometimes used now. (Redrawn with permission of the Physiological Society.)

Factors affecting contractility

A change in contractility can take place as a result of the action of various factors affecting the myocyte (Fig. 2.50). The energy of contraction is affected by other variables in addition to that of initial fibre length (Starling mechanism; Fig. 2.51). The term inotropic is also used to denote the contractility of the heart. Positive inotropes (increased contractility) include:

- Sympathetic stimulation. Noradrenaline from sympathetic nerves binds to β_1-receptors on myocytes and increases intracellular Ca^{2+} by cyclic adenosine monophosphate (cAMP)-activated protein kinase A and G-protein linked Ca^{2+} channels. This increases the force of contraction and shortens systole.
- Plasma Ca^{2+}. Increases in plasma Ca^{2+} result in increased sarcoplasmic Ca^{2+} in the myocytes.
- pH.
- Increased temperature.
- Drugs: cardiac glycosides—digoxin, ouabain; β-agonists—adrenaline, isoprenaline; and most antiarrhythmics.

Negative inotropes include:
- Disease (e.g. ischaemia, hypoxia).
- Acidity.

- Drugs: β-blockers (e.g. propranolol), Ca^{2+}-channel blockers (e.g. verapamil), barbiturates, and most anaesthetic agents.

Venous return, central venous pressure, and cardiac output

Venous return (VR) depends on the mean circulatory pressure (P_{mc}), right atrial pressure (P_{ra}) and venous resistance (R_v) according to the following formula:

$$VR = (P_{mc} - P_{ra})/R_v$$

Right atrial pressure is equivalent to the central venous pressure. The mean circulatory pressure is experimentally derived, and is the pressure that would result throughout the circulatory system if the heart were to stop beating. It is determined principally by the blood volume and the degree of sympathetic activation (Fig. 2.52). The effect of sympathetic activation is to increase the 'tightness' with which blood is constrained within the circulatory system, but this should not be confused with TPR, as this is a separate and distinct variable.

The equation is the equivalent of the previous description of arterial blood flow, i.e. flow (venous return) is equal to the pressure gradient between the central veins and the systemic circulation divided by the resistance. In health, any changes are

29

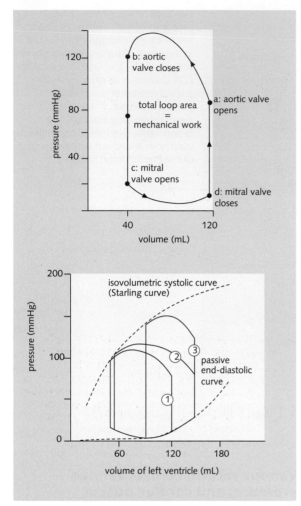

Fig. 2.49 Pressure–volume loops. (1, normal state; 2, increased end-diastolic volume (EDV) leads to increased stroke volume (SV) if arterial pressure is constant; 3, increased EDV and increased AP result in a decreased SV.) The end-systolic points of the loops produce the Starling curve so long as the contractility remains constant.

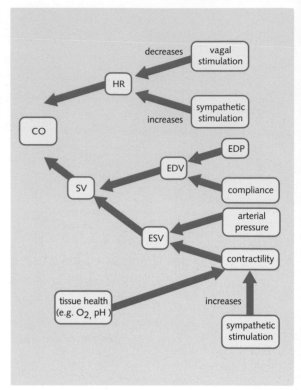

Fig. 2.50 Summary of the factors affecting cardiac output. (CO, cardiac output; EDP, end-diastolic pressure; EDV, end-diastolic volume; HR, heart rate; ESV, end-systolic volume; SV, stroke volume.)

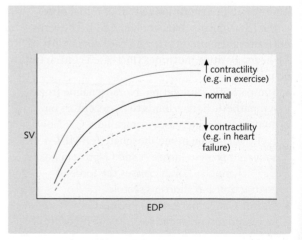

Fig. 2.51 Contractility and the Starling curve. Changes in contractility are characterized by upward (positively inotropic) and downward (negatively inotropic) displacement of the Starling curve. (EDP, end-diastolic pressure; SV, stroke volume.)

automatically compensated. For example, an increased right atrial pressure leads to reduced venous return, but it also leads to an increased output by Starling's law. This will then reduce the right atrial pressure, restoring equilibrium. There may be a transient discrepancy between venous return and cardiac output (as strictly defined), but remember that compensation occurs automatically. If the right atrial pressure remains raised, increased sympathetic activity will increase the mean filling pressure to compensate, producing a new equilibrium with a higher CVP and a higher cardiac output.

The effects of disease and resulting compensatory changes are shown in Fig. 2.53. In right-sided heart disease, where myocardial function is compromised

and right atrial pressure is persistently raised, the body compensates by increasing sympathetic drive and retaining fluid to increase blood volume (Fig.

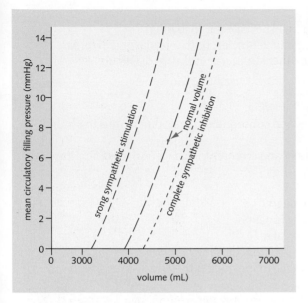

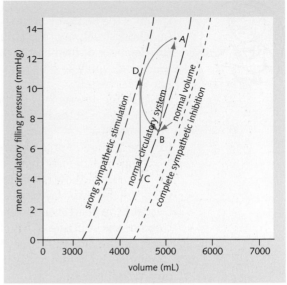

Fig. 2.52 The effects of volume and sympathetic activation on the mean circulatory filling pressure (P_{mc}). The mean filling pressure depends on the degree of filling (volume) and the stiffness of the compartment, often referred to as the tone. The reciprocal of the stiffness is called capacitance, compliance, or distensibility. The tone is increased by sympathetic stimulation, which shifts the curve to the left (vasoconstriction/venoconstriction) so that there is a higher filling pressure for a given volume. (Redrawn with permission from Guyton & Hall, 1995.)

Fig. 2.53 Examples of compensatory changes in mean circulatory filling pressure in disease. Compensatory changes in chronic heart disease (A), where volume increases and sympathetic stimulation increases mean filling pressure. Treatment is to counter these changes and unload the heart (B). In haemorrhagic shock (C), the blood loss is countered by sympathetic activation (D) (see Fig. 2.54).

2.53 A). A common treatment for this situation is nitrate, which relaxes the system as indicated in Fig. 2.53 B. In hypovolaemic shock, a reduction in blood volume is also associated with sympathetic activation (Fig. 2.53 C, D). The effects of the changes in hypovolaemic shock on cardiac function are shown in Fig. 2.54.

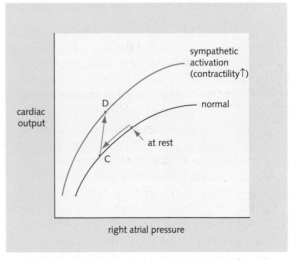

Fig. 2.54 Cardiac function curve showing the changes in haemorrhagic shock. Fluid loss causes a fall in cardiac filling (C), reducing right atrial pressure. Cardiac output will then fall, but increased sympathetic activity will increase contractility (moving the Starling curve upward and to the left) while also causing venoconstriction which will increase venous return and hence raise right atrial pressure.

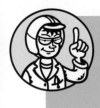

Venous return = Right heart input & output = Pulmonary blood flow = Left heart input & output = Systemic blood flow BECAUSE THEY ARE ALL **IN SERIES**

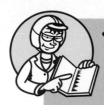

- Describe the anatomy of the heart, especially the following:
  (a) Gross structure of the atrium and ventricles, both internal and external.
  (b) Relations of the heart to the other structures in the mediastinum.
  (c) Blood supply and drainage.
  (d) Great vessels.
- Describe the embryology of the following:
  (a) The fusion of the heart tubes and subsequent development into the four chambers.
  (b) The formation of the interatrial and interventricular septa, including the congenital defects that may arise.
  (c) How the outflow tracts develop.
- What are the tissue layers of the heart?
- Describe the heart skeleton and its function.
- Describe the structure of a typical valve.
- What are the different myocytes, and how do they differ?
- Draw a basic diagram of a contractile myocyte and the arrangement with neighbouring cells.
- Sketch the internal structure of a myocyte, including myofibrils.
- Define the resting membrane potential and the factors that influence it.
- Sketch the action potential produced in the different cells of the myocardium, and explain the contribution of the different ion channels.
- What is the pacemaker potential, and how is it generated?
- Explain the role of Ca^{2+} in excitation–contraction coupling.
- What are the four phases of the cardiac cycle?
- What are the pressure changes during these cycles? Sketch the ventricular pressure–volume loop.
- Describe how jugular venous pressure changes with the events of the cardiac cycle.
- Sketch the conduction pathway.
- Define the terms cardiac output (CO), stroke volume (SV), stroke work (SW), heart rate (HR), end-diastolic volume (EDV), end-diastolic pressure (EDP), end-systolic pressure, central venous pressure (CVP), venous return (VR), total peripheral resistance (TPR), and contractility.
- State Starling's law of the heart. What is its physiological significance?
- Draw a ventricular function curve, and show how it can be changed by disease.
- Give an example of an inotropic agent, and describe the physiological factors that affect contractility.

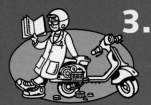

3. Structure and Function of the Vessels

Organization of the vessels

Classification of the vessels
The circulatory system is composed of vessels designed for:
- Conductance.
- Resistance.
- Exchange.
- Capacitance.

Conductance
These are low-resistance vessels, which are arteries with predominantly elastic walls. Their role is delivery of blood to more distal vessels, although they also have a small resistance role.

Resistance
These vessels are the terminal arteries and arterioles, and they are the main resistance to blood flow.

Resistance vessels act to control local blood flow. Dilatation of these vessels lowers resistance and increases blood flow (vasodilatation). Constriction of these vessels increases resistance and decreases blood flow (vasoconstriction). They can, therefore, influence the exchange vessels by governing the flow that reaches them.

Exchange
These vessels are the numerous capillaries that have very thin walls. This optimizes their function, which is to allow rapid transfer between blood and tissues. They also contribute some resistance to flow.

Capacitance
These vessels are thin-walled, low-resistance venules and veins. They act as a variable reservoir of blood and contain almost two thirds of the blood volume. These veins are innervated by venoconstrictor fibres which, when stimulated, can displace the blood into the heart.

Vasculature
The vasculature (Fig. 3.1) is classified anatomically into:
- Elastic arteries (e.g. aorta and common carotids).
- Muscular arteries (e.g. coronary, cerebral, and popliteal arteries).
- Arterioles.
- Capillaries.
- Postcapillary venules.
- Muscular venules.
- Veins.

The main function of the arteries and arterioles is to deliver blood to the capillaries. In the capillaries, exchange with and filtration into the interstitial fluid takes place. Fluid and metabolites return to the heart through veins and lymphatic vessels. Veins return blood to the heart and the lymphatic system returns excess filtrate to the blood.

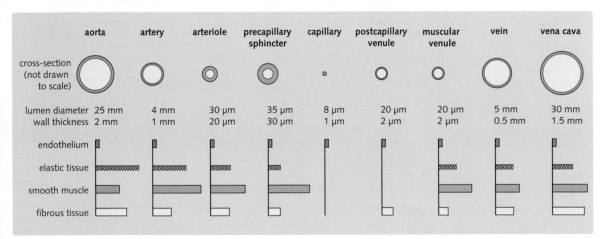

Fig. 3.1 Vessels of the circulation. (Adapted with permission from Burton AC, *Physiol Rev.* **34**: 619, 1954.)

Anatomy of the circulatory system

The anatomy of the circulatory system is shown in Figs 3.2–3.14.

Conductance vessels like the aorta also have a role in maintaining blood pressure in diastole. The systolic pressure wave is partially absorbed by elastic expansion, which is released in diastole.

Development of the circulation

The vasculature develops from the angioblastic cords of mesoderm. The aortic ends of the primitive heart tube become the aortic arches and dorsal aortae. The aortic arches develop into the great arteries of the neck and thorax, whereas the dorsal aortae produce the following branches:

- Ventral branches (derived from the remnants of the vitelline arteries). These supply the gastrointestinal tract.
- Lateral branches. These supply retroperitoneal structures (e.g. kidneys).
- Intersegmental branches. These supply the rest of the body.

Fig. 3.2 Arteries of the thorax.

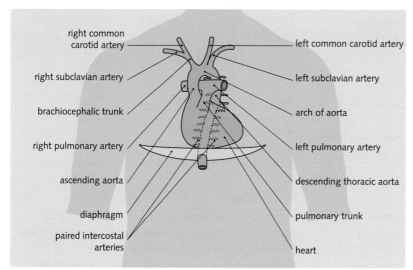

Fig. 3.3 Veins of the thorax.

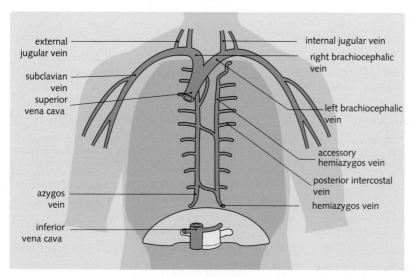

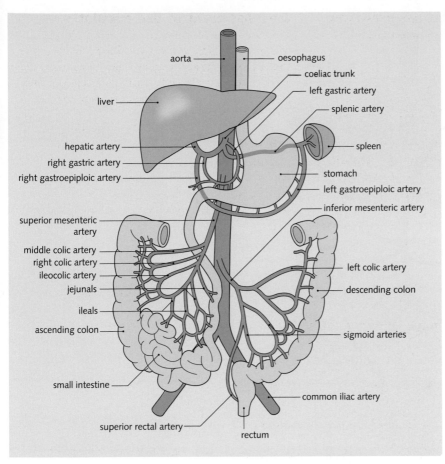

Fig. 3.4 Arteries of the abdomen.

Figure labels: aorta, oesophagus, coeliac trunk, left gastric artery, splenic artery, liver, spleen, hepatic artery, right gastric artery, right gastroepiploic artery, stomach, left gastroepiploic artery, inferior mesenteric artery, superior mesenteric artery, middle colic artery, right colic artery, ileocolic artery, jejunals, ileals, ascending colon, left colic artery, descending colon, sigmoid arteries, small intestine, common iliac artery, superior rectal artery, rectum

The paired dorsal aortae connect to the umbilical arteries, which carry blood to the placenta. The venous system consists of three components, which are initially paired:

- Cardinal system. This drains the head, neck, body wall, and limbs.
- Vitelline veins. These drain the yolk sac.
- Umbilical veins. These carry blood from the placenta to the embryo.

Initially, the venous system drains into the sinus horns, but eventually it drains into the venae cavae and right atrium. In general, it is the right-sided veins that persist while the left-sided veins regress during gestation, and so systemic venous drainage is via the vena cava to the right side of the heart. However, it is the left umbilical vein that persists while the right umbilical vein disappears.

Within the liver, the vitelline system forms the ductus venosus, which shunts blood from the umbilical vein directly into the inferior vena cava during gestation. This is vital, as it allows oxygenated blood to enter the right atrium of the heart, pass predominantly through the foramen ovale and then be pumped around the fetus (Fig. 3.15).

The foramen ovale enables the oxygenated blood in the right atrium to pass into the left atrium and reach the systemic circulation.

The ductus arteriosus develops from the sixth aortic arch. It connects the pulmonary arteries to the descending aorta. This allows oxygenated blood pumped into the pulmonary arteries to enter the systemic circulation (because the lungs are not functional during gestation, there is no need for a large pulmonary circulation). The ductus is kept open during fetal life by circulating prostaglandins.

The head receives a preferential blood supply so if there is a decrease in umbilical artery supply the head will continue to receive an adequate blood supply at the expense of the rest of the body (i.e. the head grows but the body does not).

Deoxygenated blood returns to the placenta through the umbilical arteries, which connect to the aorta.

Fig. 3.5 Veins of the abdomen.

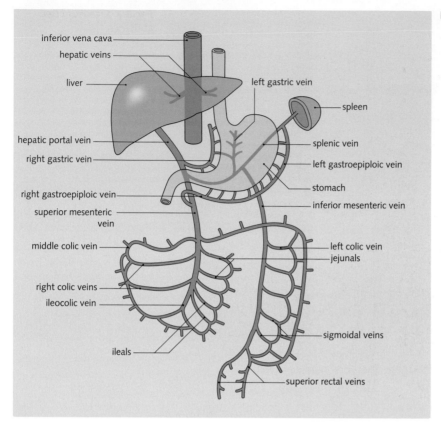

Fig. 3.6 Vessels of the pelvis.

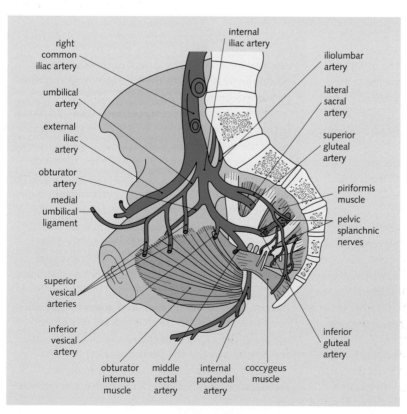

Fig. 3.7 Arteries of the neck and head.

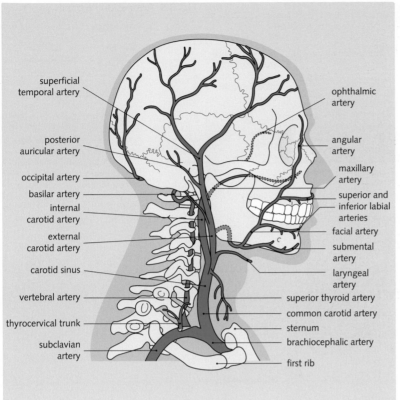

superficial temporal artery

posterior auricular artery

occipital artery

basilar artery

internal carotid artery

external carotid artery

carotid sinus

vertebral artery

thyrocervical trunk

subclavian artery

ophthalmic artery

angular artery

maxillary artery

superior and inferior labial arteries

facial artery

submental artery

laryngeal artery

superior thyroid artery

common carotid artery

sternum

brachiocephalic artery

first rib

Fig. 3.8 Veins of the neck and head.

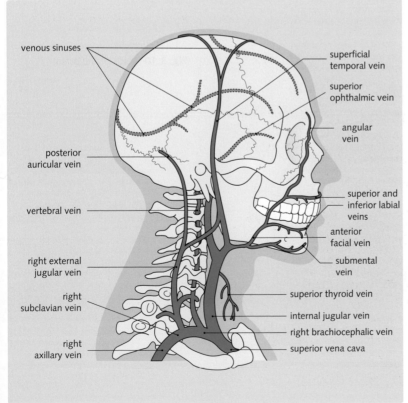

venous sinuses

posterior auricular vein

vertebral vein

right external jugular vein

right subclavian vein

right axillary vein

superficial temporal vein

superior ophthalmic vein

angular vein

superior and inferior labial veins

anterior facial vein

submental vein

superior thyroid vein

internal jugular vein

right brachiocephalic vein

superior vena cava

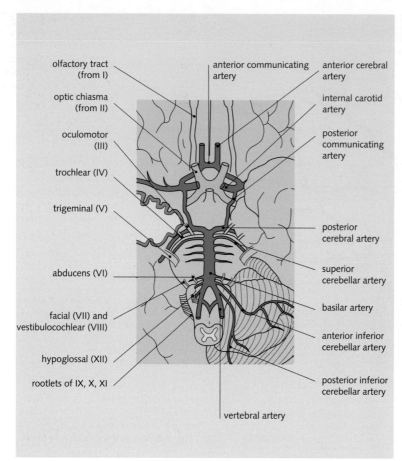

Fig. 3.9 Arteries of the brain.

olfactory tract
(from I)

optic chiasma
(from II)

oculomotor
(III)

trochlear (IV)

trigeminal (V)

abducens (VI)

facial (VII) and
vestibulocochlear (VIII)

hypoglossal (XII)

rootlets of IX, X, XI

anterior communicating
artery

anterior cerebral
artery

internal carotid
artery

posterior
communicating
artery

posterior
cerebral artery

superior
cerebellar artery

basilar artery

anterior inferior
cerebellar artery

posterior inferior
cerebellar artery

vertebral artery

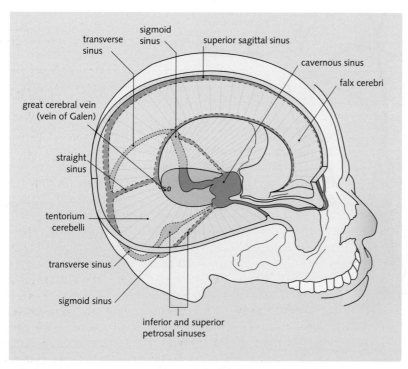

Fig. 3.10 Veins of the brain.

transverse
sinus

sigmoid
sinus

superior sagittal sinus

cavernous sinus

falx cerebri

great cerebral vein
(vein of Galen)

straight
sinus

tentorium
cerebelli

transverse sinus

sigmoid sinus

inferior and superior
petrosal sinuses

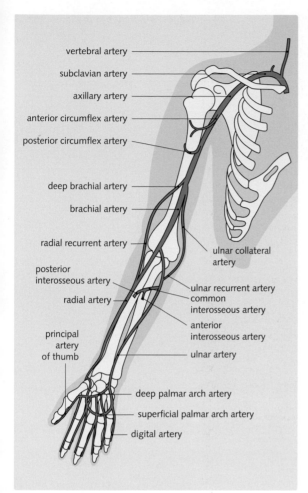

Fig. 3.11 Arteries of the upper limbs.

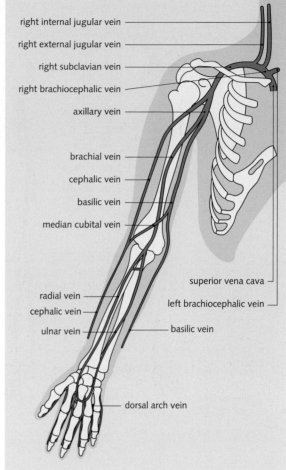

Fig. 3.12 Veins of the upper limbs.

Circulatory adaptations at birth

A series of changes convert the single system of blood flow around the fetus into dual systems at birth.

Blood flow in the umbilical vessels drastically declines in the 3–4 minutes after birth because of:

- Compression of the cord.
- Vasoconstriction in response to cold, mechanical stimuli, or catecholamines.

At birth, the pulmonary vascular resistance falls rapidly because:

- The mechanical effect of ventilation opens the constricted alveolar vessels.
- Raising P_{O_2} and lowering P_{CO_2} causes vasodilatation of the pulmonary vessels.

This produces an increase in the pulmonary blood flow.

The sudden cessation of umbilical blood flow and the opening of the pulmonary system causes a change in the pressure balance in the atria. There is a pressure drop in the right atrium and a pressure rise in the left atrium (caused by an increased pulmonary venous return to the left atrium). This changes the pressure gradient across the atria and forces the flexible septum primum against the rigid septum secundum, closing the foramen ovale. These two septa will fuse together after about 3 months.

The ductus venosus closes soon after birth (Figs 3.16 and 3.17). The mechanism is unclear, but it may involve prostaglandin inhibition.

The closure is not vital to life, as the umbilical vein no longer carries any blood.

The ductus arteriosus closes 1–8 days after birth. It is thought that as the pulmonary circulation fills, the pressure drop in the pulmonary trunk causes blood to flow from the aorta into the pulmonary

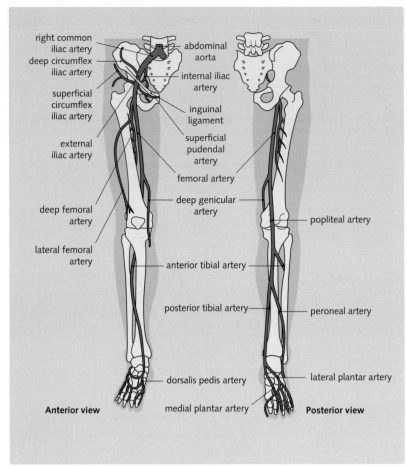

Fig. 3.13 Arteries of the lower limbs.

right common iliac artery
deep circumflex iliac artery
superficial circumflex iliac artery
external iliac artery
deep femoral artery
lateral femoral artery
abdominal aorta
internal iliac artery
inguinal ligament
superficial pudendal artery
femoral artery
deep genicular artery
popliteal artery
anterior tibial artery
posterior tibial artery
peroneal artery
dorsalis pedis artery
lateral plantar artery
medial plantar artery

Anterior view   **Posterior view**

trunk through the ductus arteriosus. This blood is oxygenated and the increase in P_{O_2} causes the smooth muscle in the wall of the ductus to constrict. This obstructs flow in the ductus arteriosus.

Eventually, the intima of the ductus arteriosus thickens—complete obliteration of the ductus results in the formation of the ligamentum arteriosum, which attaches the pulmonary trunk to the aorta.

Congenital vascular abnormalities

Many circulatory anomalies can develop, but few of these conditions cause any problems. Those that do include:

- Patent ductus arteriosus. This is when the ductus arteriosus fails to close.
- Coarctation of the aorta. This is abnormal stenotic thickening of the aorta that affects systemic blood flow.
- Persistent patent foramen ovale. This is caused by a failure of fusion of the septum primum and

secundum, leading to a permanent shunt between the atria.

Further information on these may be found in Chapter 5.

The components of a vessel wall reflect that vessel's function. For example, if a vessel wall contains many elastic fibres, it will be more compliant than other vessels and better suited to act as a conductance vessel.

Structure and histology

A blood vessel has an endothelium surrounded by three main layers (or tunicae). These are termed the intima, media, and adventitia. Fig. 3.18 shows the layers of a typical vessel.

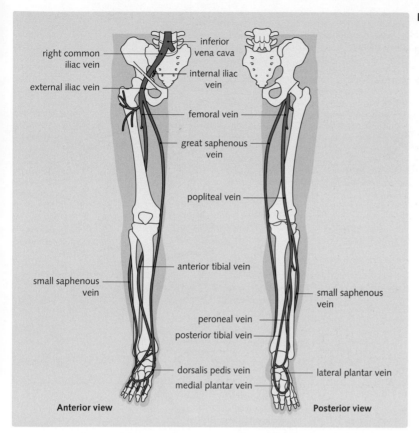

Fig. 3.14 Veins of the lower limbs.

Anterior view

Posterior view

Fig. 3.15 Fetal blood pathway.

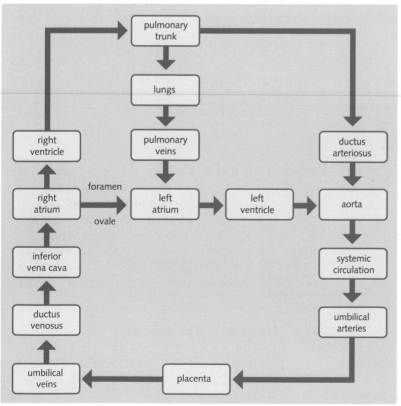

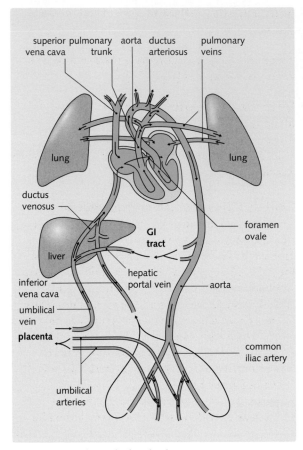

Fig. 3.16 Circulation before birth.

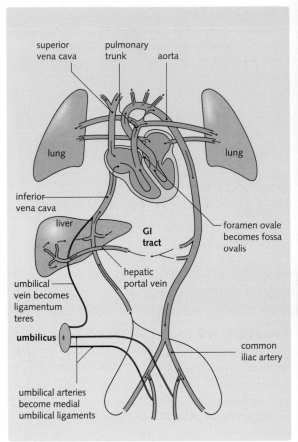

Fig. 3.17 Circulation after birth. Note the closure of the foramen ovale, ductus arteriosus, ductus venosus, and umbilical vessels closing off the fetal shunts.

Fig. 3.18 Cross-section of a generic vessel showing the order of the layers.

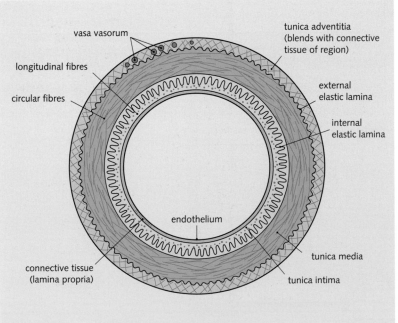

Arteries and veins

An elastic artery consists of concentric layers of elastic and smooth muscle, whereas a muscular artery has prominent muscular media, with internal and external elastic laminae. In contrast a vein has a thin media. Fig. 3.19 shows the structure of an elastic artery, a muscular artery, and a vein.

Capillary

The structure of a capillary is shown in Fig. 3.20.

Lymphatic vessel

The structure of a lymphatic capillary is shown in Fig. 3.21.

Vascular endothelium and smooth muscle

Functions of endothelial cells

Endothelial cells (see Fig. 3.35) are involved in:
- Transportation of substances between interstitium and plasma.
- Providing a friction-free surface.
- Regulation of clotting.
- Inflammatory responses.
- Control of vascular tone.

Some of these functions require the secretion of a variety of substances (Fig. 3.22).

Vascular smooth muscle
Structure
The structure of smooth muscle is shown in Fig. 3.23. A mass of smooth muscle functions as if it were a single unit.

Contraction of vascular smooth muscle
Contraction is initiated by a rise in intracellular Ca^{2+}. This leads to an actin–myosin interaction, which causes shortening and tension. The process differs from that of the myocardium in the following ways:
- Myosin light chain phosphorylation. Unlike skeletal or cardiac muscle, the myosin in vascular smooth muscle only becomes active if its light chains are phosphorylated. The enzyme is activated by a calcium–calmodulin complex, which is dependent on a rise in intracellular Ca^{2+} for its formation.
- Sustained actin–myosin interactions enable vascular smooth muscle to maintain tension for

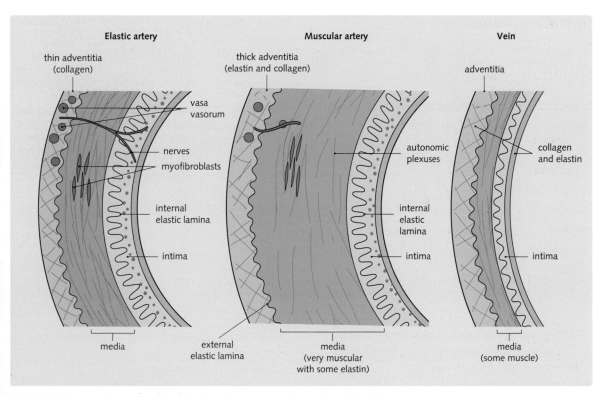

Fig. 3.19 Cross-sections of walls of elastic arteries, muscular arteries, and veins.

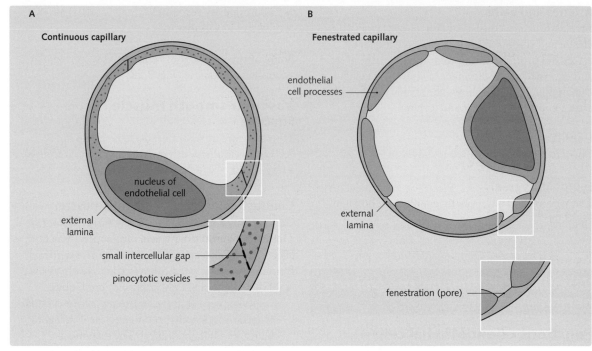

Fig. 3.20 Cross-sections of capillaries with continuous and fenestrated walls. Continuous capillary walls are less permeable than fenestrated capillary walls. (Redrawn with permission from Stevens and Lowe, 1997.)

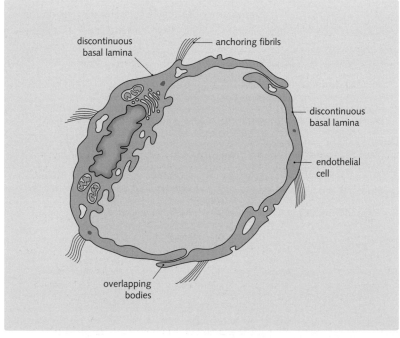

Fig. 3.21 Cross-section of a lymph capillary. Lymph capillaries only allow flow into the lumen but not out. Overlapping endothelial cells operate as one way valves to accomplish this. The anchoring filaments connect the endothelial cells to the surrounding tissue. When surrounding tissues are swollen with excess interstitial fluid (e.g. in inflammation) the filaments pull the endothelial cells apart to increase lymphatic flow. The discontinuous basal lamina (basement membrane) also allows greater movement of fluids and solutes.

0.3% of the energy needed by skeletal muscle. The actin–myosin interactions are long-lasting because of slow myosin kinetics.

- Sensitivity to intracellular Ca^{2+}. Chemical factors can alter the relationship between cytoplasmic Ca^{2+} and contractile force (i.e. the sensitivity of the contractile apparatus to Ca^{2+} can be changed). The cytoplasmic Ca^{2+} concentration and the resting membrane potential are dependent upon the state of

Secreted factors and their functions	
Factor secreted	**Function**
Structural components	To form the basal lamina
Prostacyclin	Vasodilatation; inhibits platelet aggregation
Nitric oxide	Vasodilatation; inhibits platelet adhesion and aggregation
Angiotensin converting enzyme	Converts angiotensin I to II; degrades bradykinin and serotonin
Platelet activating factor	Activates platelets and neutrophils
Tissue plasminogen activator (tPA)	Regulates fibrinolysis
Thromboplastin	Promotes coagulation
Von Willebrand's factor	Promotes platelet adhesion and clotting

Fig. 3.22 Secreted factors from endothelial cells and their functions.

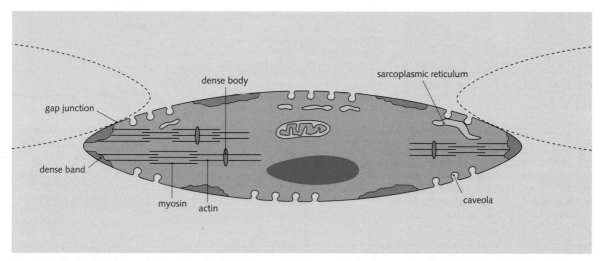

Fig. 3.23 Structure of smooth muscle cell. The actin–myosin filaments have been magnified. (Adapted from Levick R. *Introducing Cardiovascular Physiology*. Butterworth–Heinemann, 1995. Reproduced by permission of Edward Arnold Ltd.)

ion-conducting channels (K^+, Ca^{2+}, and Cl^- channels).

Effect of sympathetic innervation

Fig. 3.24 shows the mechanism of sympathetic innervation.

Vascular smooth muscle relaxation

Vascular smooth muscle relaxation can be brought about by three (or, possibly, four) different mechanisms. Each mechanism relies upon reducing intracellular Ca^{2+}:

- Hyperpolarization. Hyperpolarizing the resting membrane reduces the number of open Ca^{2+} channels, leading to a decrease in intracellular Ca^{2+} concentration and relaxation. Hyperpolarization is caused by hypoxia, acidosis, calcitonin-gene-related peptide, and drugs (e.g. diazoxide, cromakalim, pinacidil).
- Cyclic adenosine monophosphate (cAMP)-mediated vasodilatation (Fig. 3.25).
- Cyclic guanosine monophosphate (cGMP)-mediated vasodilatation (Fig. 3.26).
- Sensitivity to intracellular Ca^{2+} is probably another cause of relaxation. This lowers the sensitivity of the contractile apparatus to the cytoplasmic Ca^{2+}. This makes the contraction weaker for a given concentration of Ca^{2+} and causes dilatation.

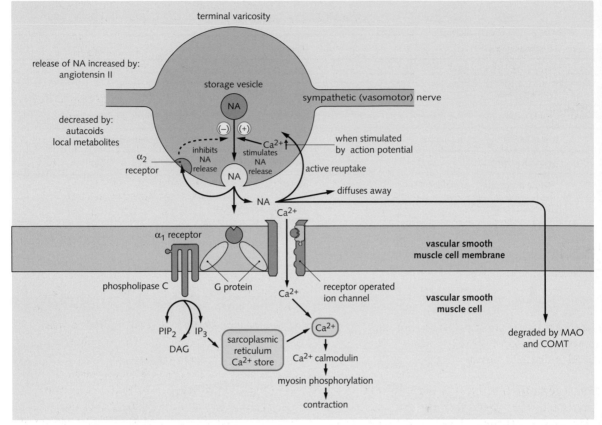

Fig. 3.24 Release of noradrenaline (NA) from a sympathetic junction and its effect on the vascular smooth muscle (VSM) cell. Sympathetic stimulation results in the release of NA from the sympathetic terminal varicosities. NA acts on α_1-receptors on the VSM cells. This results in an increase in intracellular Ca^{2+} by directly opening Ca^{2+} channels and via a second messenger system releasing Ca^{2+} from the sarcoplasmic reticulum. It is the increase of intracellular Ca^{2+} that brings about contraction. (AP, action potential; COMT, catechol O-methyltransferase; DAG, diacylglycerol; IP$_3$, inositol triphosphate; MAO, monoamine oxidase; PIP$_2$, phosphatidyl inositol bisphosphate.)

Isoprenaline may work in this way as well as with cAMP-mediated vasodilatation.

Haemodynamics in arteries and veins

Haemodynamics in arteries

In normal arteries and veins, there is laminar flow (Fig. 3.27). Turbulent flow occurs in the ventricles.

Noradrenaline contracts smooth muscle, whereas nitric oxide relaxes smooth muscle (NO = no contraction).

Single-file flow occurs in capillaries. Although this is a simplistic view it is sufficient for most basic purposes.

Pulse waveform

The difference between systolic and diastolic pressure is termed the pulse pressure. The pressure wave created by ventricular ejection depends upon:

- Stroke volume.
- Heart rate.
- Elasticity of the arterial wall.
- Peripheral resistance.
- Blood volume.

The mean arterial pressure is the arterial pressure averaged over time. Mean arterial pressure is not just midway between diastolic and systolic pressure. The time spent in diastole is longer than that spent in systole (Fig. 3.28). Thus, mean arterial pressure is

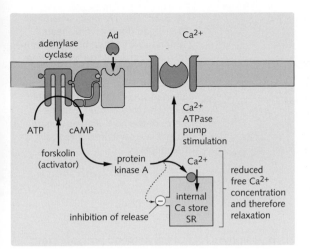

Fig. 3.25 cAMP-mediated vasodilatation as shown by the action of adrenaline (Ad). (ATP, adenosine triphosphate; SR, sarcoplasmic reticulum.)

1. Wrap the cuff around upper arm of the patient, who should be sitting or lying during the procedure.
2. Palpate the radial or brachial artery and inflate the cuff until the pulse is no longer palpable.
3. Auscultate the brachial artery at the medial side of the antecubital fossa with a stethoscope. No sound should be heard.
4. Gradually lower the cuff pressure until a dull tapping sound is heard. The measurement taken at this time is the systolic pressure.
5. Further lowering of the cuff pressure results in louder sounds until the sounds suddenly become quieter, but still present. The measurement taken at this time is the diastolic pressure.

Normal blood pressure

Normal blood pressure for a healthy adult male at rest is 120/80 mmHg. However, this value can vary because of many factors, and these must be taken into account when assessing a patient's blood pressure:

- Ageing causes an increase in blood pressure because of decreased arterial compliance caused by arteriosclerosis. As a rough rule, systolic pressure should be equal to 100 mmHg plus age in years.
- During sleep, blood pressure falls because of the body's decreased metabolic demands.

closer to diastolic pressure. It is commonly approximated as one third of the pulse pressure added to diastolic pressure.

Measurement of arterial blood pressure

Arterial blood pressure can be measured directly by using invasive catheters. However, it is usual practice in most patients to measure blood pressure indirectly using a sphygmomanometer.

The sphygmomanometer is used as follows:

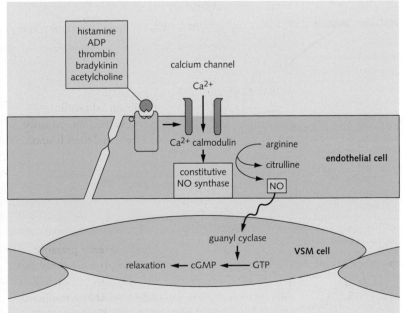

Fig. 3.26 cGMP-mediated vasodilatation as shown by action of vasoactive mediators adenosine diphosphate; GTP, guanosine triphosphate; NO, nitric oxide; VSM cell, vascular smooth muscle cell.)

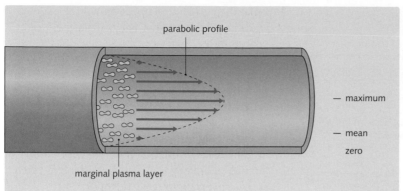

Fig. 3.27 The dynamics of laminar flow. Blood flows as if in sheets (laminae) with blood being faster in the middle than at the sides, where friction slows flow. The dashed line indicates the parabolic profile of the different speeds across the vessel. Cells tend to accumulate in the centre of the flow, leaving a marginal plasma layer with fewer red cells at the periphery.

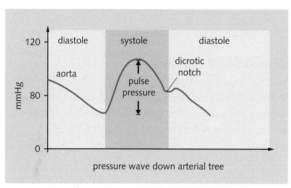

Fig. 3.28 Pulse waveform. The dicrotic notch is caused by closure of the aortic valve.

- Heavy dynamic exercise increases blood pressure because of increased cardiac output. However, the increase in blood pressure is less than 30% because of decreased total peripheral resistance.
- Heavy static exercise greatly increases blood pressure (possibly, by more than 30%) because of the exercise pressor response.
- Anger, sexual excitement, and stress increase blood pressure, all because of sympathetically mediated responses.

Other factors that may cause changes in blood pressure include:
- Respiration. In the young, mean arterial pressure falls by a small amount during inspiration because of a transient fall in stroke volume.
- Pregnancy. Blood pressure falls gradually in the first trimester, reaching a minimum in the second trimester, and then rises to normal in the third trimester.
- Physiological processes. For example, the Valsalva manoeuvre and the diving reflex.
- Pathological processes. For example, shock, haemorrhage, and heart failure.

There is a physiological fall in blood pressure from the major arteries through the vascular tree. Note that the largest pressure drop is at arteriolar level, the site of the main resistance to blood flow (Fig. 3.29).

Blood flow and velocity

Blood flow is defined as the volume of blood that flows through a given tissue in a given time. For the whole body, this must equal the cardiac output. Ohm's law states:

Flow = (Pressure difference)/resistance $(I = V/R)$

Hence, the determinants of flow are the blood pressure within a vessel (see above) and the resistance to flow within the vessel (see below).

Velocity of blood flow

The velocity of blood flow is inversely related to the total cross-sectional area (Fig. 3.30). The branching

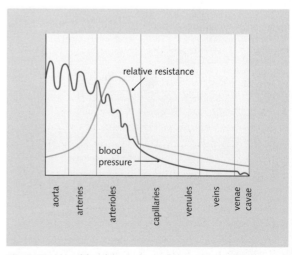

Fig. 3.29 How blood pressure and vascular resistance change across the vascular system. Pressure in the arterial side and in the great veins varies with the cardiac cycle.

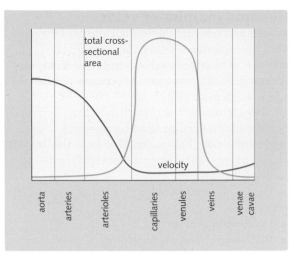

Fig. 3.30 Total cross-sectional area and velocity within the different anatomical classifications of vessels. Velocity in the arterial side actually varies with the cardiac cycle, the mean velocity is shown.

Remember Poiseuille's law only applies to laminar (smooth) flow in vessels. Constrictions or high systolic pressure can increase the velocity, creating turbulence (the opposite of laminar flow). In most cases, turbulent flow creates noise, which is the basis for auscultating bruits from arterial narrowing and Korotkow sounds when measuring blood pressure.

Blood flow through vessels can be compared to water flow through pipes (i.e. ignoring the effect of blood cells). If a hose pipe is narrowed, water flows more slowly (try it!); similarly, as blood vessels become narrower, flow is reduced (so long as other factors remain constant). A blood vessel may be narrowed by disease (e.g. atheromatous changes), reducing the flow.

nature of the circulatory system means that the total cross-sectional area of the capillaries is much greater than that of the arteries or veins. This reduces velocity in the capillaries.

Vascular resistance
Poiseuille's law
Poiseuille determined that resistance (R) to the steady laminar flow of a fluid through a tube is proportional to the length of the tube (l), viscosity of the fluid (η), and inversely proportional to the radius of the tube to the fourth power (r^4). He stated:

$$R = 8\,\eta l/\pi r^4$$

Using Ohm's law (I = V/R) we can derive:

$$\text{Flow} = (\text{Pressure difference}) \times \pi\,r^4/8\,\eta l$$

From these equations we can explain the resistance element of Fig. 3.29:
- Total resistance in the vasculature is greatest in the arterioles, through a combination of their length and reduced radius without a significant change in total cross-sectional area.
- Capillary resistance is less than arteriolar resistance because capillaries are shorter (0.5 mm), large numbers of capillaries occur in parallel, and they have single-file flow rather than laminar flow.
- Total resistance is dependent upon smooth muscle tension, which controls the arteriolar radius.

Vasoconstriction and vasodilatation
Constriction of the vascular smooth muscle will cause an arteriole to narrow. This is termed vasoconstriction. Vasodilatation is the term used when smooth muscle relaxes and expands the lumen of the vessel. Vasodilatation will increase the radius of the vessel and lower its resistance. This will increase blood flow through it. Vasoconstriction will have the opposite effect, narrowing the vessel, increasing resistance, and decreasing blood flow.

Laplace's law states that the tension in the wall of a vessel needed to restore a drop in pressure across its wall is dependent upon the radius of the vessel. Or, at a given blood pressure, the tension in the wall fibres increases with the radius. Conversely, at a given radius, the tension increases with blood pressure.

This helps to explain vasoconstriction and vasodilatation. There are two components to wall tension:
- Active tension (from the vascular smooth muscle).

- Passive tension (from connective tissue—collagen and elastin).

Constriction of the smooth muscle increases active tension and decreases the radius. Assuming that the blood pressure remains constant, Laplace's law states that the net wall tension must decrease. This decrease is brought about by a fall in passive tension. That is, an equilibrium is reached between active tension, passive tension, and the internal distending pressure of the blood.

Variations in this tension bring about vasoconstriction and vasodilatation.

Blood viscosity

Viscosity, defined as 'lack of slipperiness' by Newton, is the measure of the internal friction within a moving fluid. According to Poiseuille's law, resistance is proportional to viscosity. So, viscosity of the blood plays a major role in determining resistance and, therefore, blood flow.

Plasma viscosity is increased by the presence of proteins (mainly albumins and globulins). Blood viscosity is affected by plasma viscosity, but it is the haematocrit (the percentage of red cells in the blood volume) that is the main determinant.

Haematocrit is at an optimal level for oxygen delivery. An elevated haematocrit increases the carriage of oxygen, but it raises viscosity, impeding flow and increasing cardiac work.

A normal haematocrit value of 47% makes blood viscosity about four times that of water, as measured in a special wide-bore viscometer. However, viscosity *in vivo* is affected by the radius of the vessels and the flow rate.

Viscosity is also affected by physiological or pathological processes, such as polycythaemia (raised haematocrit) or myeloma (cancer of immunoglobulin-secreting cells).

Polycythaemia is caused by a physiological adaptation to chronic hypoxia or a myeloproliferative disease resulting in increased red blood cell production by the bone marrow (polycythaemia rubra vera). Viscosity and, therefore, resistance are increased, leading to hypertension and sluggish blood flow. Thrombosis may occur.

In myeloma, there is an increased production of immunoglobulin. Immunoglobulins can cause red blood cells to agglutinate, which leads to increased blood viscosity and increased resistance. This impairs perfusion, especially in cold fingers and toes, and ischaemia/necrosis can result.

Haemodynamics of veins

Venules and veins are thin-walled, distensible vessels. They are capacitance vessels, being a variable reservoir of blood for cardiac filling. Venous blood volume depends on the venous pressure and the active wall tension (Fig. 3.31).

Active tension of the smooth muscle is controlled by sympathetic nervous stimulation, which causes venoconstriction. This pushes blood into the thoracic compartment—an important process in regulating cardiac filling pressure.

Venous pressures when supine (i.e. at heart level) are:

- 12–20 mmHg in venules.
- 8–10 mmHg in the femoral vein.
- 0–6 mmHg in the central veins and right atrium.

Although these pressures are small, resistance is also small, and the pressure is sufficient to drive blood into the right atrium.

Effect of posture and gravity

Orthostasis (the movement from supine to standing) increases blood pressure in any vessel below heart level. This is caused by the effect of gravity on the column of blood in the vessel.

Blood is prevented from flowing backwards in the veins because of the closure of venous valves. Pressure rises in the veins because blood is continually flowing into the veins from the capillaries. This will open the valves and re-establish a continuous column of blood to the heart. This means that the venous pressure in the legs increases up to 10-fold. The pressure increase will distend the venous walls and cause venous pooling in the legs.

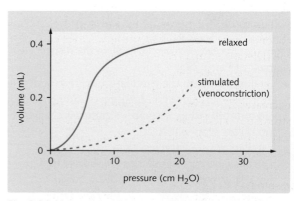

Fig. 3.31 Venous pressure curve. For a given pressure venous blood volume is greater when the venous wall muscle is relaxed than when the veins are constricted. Changes in the active wall tension can be used to displace blood into the heart.

This pooling causes a fall in central venous pressure and, therefore, cardiac filling and stroke volume. Reflex mechanisms then operate, causing vasoconstriction to try to maintain blood pressure.

In veins close to the right atrium, pressure becomes pulsatile. The pulse pressure in veins is not palpable, being small, but it is sufficient to distend the skin. This oscillation in pressure and, therefore, flow is caused by the motion of the heart and atrial activity (see Chapter 2 for more details). Venous flow in the great veins is also aided by the skeletal muscle pump and respiration.

Skeletal muscle pump

Rhythmic exercise, especially of the leg muscles, produces a pumping effect resulting in redistribution of venous blood into the central veins, maintaining central venous pressure (Fig. 3.32). This exercise also lowers distal venous pressure, producing an increased arteriovenous pressure difference, driving more blood into the working muscle; it also decreases capillary filtration pressure, thereby reducing swelling.

Incompetent venous valves will make the skeletal muscle pump ineffective. This means that the vertical column of blood is uninterrupted, which leads to a constant distending pressure. Permanent distension (varicose veins) can result.

Respiratory pump

In the central veins, flow increases during inspiration. There is a fall in intrathoracic pressure, and the diaphragm compresses the abdomen, increasing abdominal pressure.

This results in increased blood flow from the abdomen to thorax. This increases venous return to the right atrium and thereby increases right ventricular stroke volume.

However, left ventricular stroke volume decreases. This is because the pulmonary veins are stretched, and they have a greater capacitance during inspiration, which reduces left atrial filling. The opposite occurs during expiration. Overall, the output of the two ventricles is equal over the whole respiratory cycle.

Systemic blood pressure can reflect this cycle, especially in the young. It will be:
- Decreased in inspiration.
- Increased in expiration.

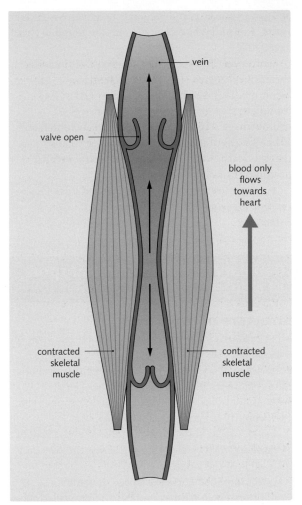

Fig. 3.32 Skeletal muscle pump. Constriction of the surrounding muscle drives the blood towards the heart. It is prevented from going the other way by the closure of venous valves.

Haemostasis and thrombosis

Haemostasis is the term used to refer to the regulation of blood clotting and the response of an injured vessel (i.e. vasoconstriction, see Chapter 4). It describes a dynamic balance between the maintenance of blood as a fluid and the production of a clot or thrombus at a site of injury. Note that the term thrombus is used to refer to an intravascular coagulation event, and not the physiological clot that forms when a vessel is broken open, e.g. by an external wound.

Clotting is initiated by endothelial cell injury, platelet activation, or activation of the plasma proteins which form the coagulation cascade (factors I–XII). The common end result is the formation of an aggregation of platelets enmeshed in cross-linked fibrin. Red and white cells may also be found in this aggregate.

Common abnormalities of haemostasis include thrombocytopenia (low platelet count) and haemophilia (heritable loss of factor VIII or IX) leading to slow coagulation and extensive haemorrhage. Hypercoagulable states include factor V Leiden (heritable mutation of factor V) and thrombocythaemia (raised platelet count) which promote thrombus formation.

For full coverage of this subject, see *Crash Course: Immunology and Haematology* and *Crash Course: Pathology*.

Capillary dynamics and transport of solutes

Structure of capillaries

Most capillaries are thin walled, with a single layer of endothelial cells on a basement membrane. Some have a second layer of cells. There is neither smooth muscle nor elastic tissue in their walls. The arrangement of the endothelial cells determines the permeability of capillaries (see Fig. 3.20).

Laplace's law states that the tension in the wall of a vessel depends on the pressure across the wall and the radius of the vessel.

Love simplified Laplace's law, to derive an equilibrium equation that applies to a thin-walled tube:

$$\text{Tension} = \Delta P \times r$$

where ΔP is pressure difference and r is vessel radius.

As capillaries have very small radii, $\Delta P \times r$ will be a small value. Therefore, the tension in the wall needed to counteract the blood pressure in the capillary will be small.

This, in combination with the massive total cross-sectional area, allows the capillaries to withstand blood pressure even though their walls are very thin.

Capillary circulation

Blood flow across the capillary bed is not constant but fluctuates (Fig. 3.33). Flow may be variable or even reversible—this is termed vasomotion.

Vasomotion is determined by the pathway through tissues, which is governed by the closure of different precapillary sphincters.

Arteriovenous anastomoses are not capillaries, as they contain smooth muscle. They do not undertake gaseous exchange. They are important in temperature regulation.

Capillary diameter may be smaller than red cell diameter, but because the red blood cells can deform they are still able to flow through. This may help gaseous exchange, as the cell walls are forced closer to the endothelium.

Starling's forces and capillary exchange of fluid

Starling's hypothesis of tissue fluid formation is a balance of two main forces: hydrostatic pressure (forcing fluid out of the capillaries) and osmotic pressure (also known as colloid oncotic pressure, absorbing fluid back into the capillaries).

Hydrostatic pressure results from the pressure of blood entering the capillaries from the arterioles. It is

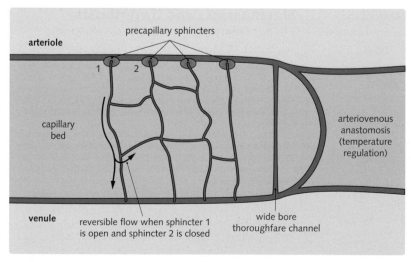

Fig. 3.33 Capillary circulation. Flow may be reversible in some vessels (vasomotion) depending on the closure of the precapillary sphincters.

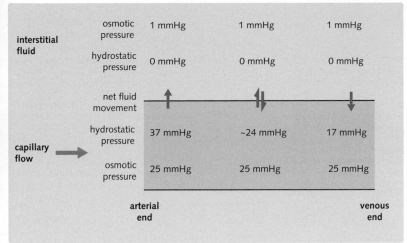

Fig. 3.34 Factors affecting fluid movement across the capillary endothelium. The fall in hydrostatic pressure across the capillary reverses the direction of fluid movement. At the arterial end, there is a net filtration pressure of (37–25) – (1–0) = 11 mmHg forcing fluid out of the capillary. At the venous end, this value becomes (17–25) – (1–0) = –9 mmHg, indicating a net filtration pressure drawing fluid back into the capillary.

typically 37 mmHg at the arterial end of the capillary and 17 mmHg at the venous end. The hydrostatic pressure of the interstitial fluid is around 0 mmHg.

Osmotic pressure is produced by the plasma proteins, because the smaller molecules can diffuse across the vessel wall, equilibrating their concentrations, but large proteins cannot. Osmotic pressure in the plasma is typically 25 mmHg, and in the interstitium is 1 mmHg.

These forces balance along most of the capillary except at the two ends. At the arterial end a net filtration of fluid occurs, whereas at the venous end a net absorption takes place (Fig. 3.34). It is also probable that more filtration occurs when the precapillary sphincter is open, and more absorption occurs when the sphincter is closed.

The amount of fluid entering and leaving the capillary is small compared with the amount of fluid moving along the capillary. The exchange of fluid:

- Plays no role in the exchange of nutrients and metabolites, which occurs by diffusion.

Capillary forces are like a seesaw. At one end, hydrostatic pressure is greater than osmotic pressure and water filters out. At the other end, osmotic pressure is greater than hydrostatic pressure and water filters in.

- Is important for determining volumes of plasma and interstitial fluid.

If conditions change, the balance between filtration and absorption will change:

- An increase in hydrostatic pressure will force fluid into the interstitial space. Oedema results if there is an accumulation of fluid in this space.
- In liver disease or severe starvation, plasma protein levels fall, decreasing osmotic pressure. This will also drive fluid into the interstitium, leading to oedema.
- Capillaries become more permeable to protein when damaged, causing a decrease in plasma osmotic pressure and leading to oedema (this process occurs, for example, in the swelling of a sprained joint).

Capillary transport mechanisms

Exchange of solutes generally occurs by diffusion down concentration gradients. The processes involved include:

- Diffusion through the endothelial cell membrane.
- Diffusion through pores and fenestrations in the cell membrane.
- Active transportation by transcytotic vesicles (Fig. 3.35).

Lipid-soluble substances (e.g. oxygen and carbon dioxide) diffuse readily through the endothelial cell membrane of the entire capillary wall.

Pores and fenestrations

Water-soluble substances (e.g. water, glucose, amino acids, ions) diffuse through the many small pores

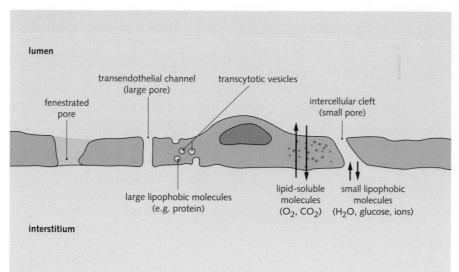

Fig. 3.35 Summary diagram of capillary transport showing the various transport mechanisms.

(radii of 4 nm) that constitute the intercellular clefts between endothelial cells. There are also a few large pores for larger molecules, especially in the liver and spleen, where the endothelium is not continuous.

Fenestrated capillaries in exocrine glands have large windows (50 nm radius), which are covered with a mesh of fibres that does not allow through molecules larger than 70 kD. This makes the capillaries more permeable to water, but prevents proteins from passing.

In the brain, the endothelial cell junctions have a complex arrangement of fibres that make them impermeable to lipophobic molecules. This comprises the blood–brain barrier, which tightly controls the neuronal environment of the brain.

Transcytotic vesicles

Some molecules (e.g. proteins) are transported across the endothelial cell by vesicles. This is an active transport process requiring energy.

Lymph and the lymphatic system

Distribution of the lymphatic tissues

Fluid and any proteins and fat globules not reabsorbed into capillaries are brought back into the blood system through the lymphatic system (Fig. 3.36). There is a network of lymphatic capillaries, ducts, and lymph nodes that unite to form the thoracic duct, which drains into the left subclavian vein.

No lymph drainage exists in the brain or eye, which have their own drainage systems—the cerebrospinal fluid and aqueous humour.

There are certain specialized areas of lymphatic tissue associated with the immune response:
- Primary lymphoid tissue—thymus and bone marrow.
- Secondary lymphoid tissue—lymph nodes, spleen, and mucosa-associated lymphoid tissue (MALT).

Further details can be found in *Crash Course: Immune, Blood, and Lymphatic Systems*.

Structure of lymph vessels

Lymph capillaries are blind ending, thin walled, and usually form a network of tubes of 10–50 μm diameter (see Fig. 3.21). These terminal lymphatics have large endothelial cell junctions, and so they are permeable to plasma proteins and other large molecules. These cell junctions may act like valves, preventing fluid moving back into the interstitium.

Lymph capillaries join together to form collecting vessels, which may contain valves to prevent backflow. Lymph vessels of this size and larger also have smooth muscle in their walls. Afferent vessels drain into a lymph node, where the fluid is presented to the immune system. Some lymph may enter the blood system at these nodes.

Efferent vessels leave the lymph node and enter the cisterna chyli, which acts as a temporary reservoir for chylomicrons from the gut. Eventually, the lymph drains into the large thoracic duct, which drains into the left subclavian vein.

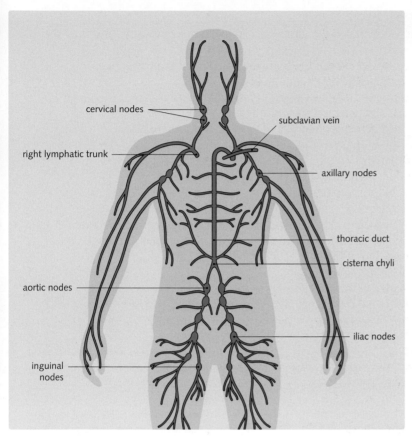

Fig. 3.36 Lymphatic drainage of the body. The lymphatics drain into the left and right subclavian veins.

Labels on figure: cervical nodes, subclavian vein, right lymphatic trunk, axillary nodes, thoracic duct, cisterna chyli, aortic nodes, iliac nodes, inguinal nodes

Fluid and proteins are driven into the lymphatic capillaries by the interstitial fluid pressure (possibly aided by lymphatic contraction creating suction). Lymph is moved along the lymphatics by smooth muscle contractions in the vessel wall, which increase with volume, and extrinsic propulsion by the skeletal muscle pump and intestinal peristalsis. Backflow is prevented by the presence of valves.

Role of the lymphatics

The role of the lymphatic system is four-fold:

- Transportation of fluid and proteins. This maintains fluid balance by returning capillary filtrate to the blood.
- Absorption and transport of fat from the gastrointestinal tract. Chylomicrons are tiny fat globules, which are absorbed into intestinal lymph vessels (lacteals).
- Presentation of foreign materials to the immune system. Phagocytosis of particles can occur in the lymph nodes.
- Circulation of lymphocytes. If the immune response is stimulated, lymphocytes can be released from lymph nodes into the lymph to be carried into the blood.

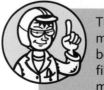

The lymphatics are the mopping up system of the body, taking up any excess filtrate and returning it to the main circulatory system. They also carry foreign antigens from the blood to cells of the immune system located in the lymph nodes.

- Describe the functional and anatomical classifications of vessels, and how the classifications differ.
- What are the main vessels of the body and their main branches?
- How does the fetal circulation change at birth?
- Describe the layers of a typical major vessel with their functions.
- List the functions of the vascular endothelium.
- What factors affect the contractility of vascular smooth muscle?
- Explain how noradrenaline brings about contraction of vascular smooth muscle.
- Explain how relaxation is brought about in vascular smooth muscle.
- Sketch the pulse waveform; what is the pulse pressure?
- Describe how to measure blood pressure.
- What is Poiseuille's law?
- Explain the basis for the changes in vascular resistance through the vascular tree. How do these changes affect blood pressure and the velocity of blood flow?
- What alters viscosity of blood?
- What affects venous flow?
- How do capillaries withstand blood pressure?
- Describe a typical capillary bed and how flow fluctuates.
- Explain Starling's capillary forces and how the movement of water varies within the capillary.
- What are the various methods of capillary transport?
- Outline the distribution of the lymph vessels in the body.
- What is the role of the lymphatic system?

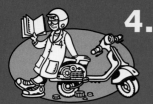

4. Control of the Cardiovascular System

Control of blood vessels

Overview of vascular control

The main function of the vasculature is to deliver metabolic requirements to the tissues of the body. Some tissues have a greater need than others (Fig. 4.1), depending on their function at a given time (e.g. muscles in exercise).

Some tissues can survive without these substrates longer than others (e.g. muscle cells can survive hypoxia for hours, whereas the brain will die within minutes).

Local control mechanisms

Local temperature

This is the main control mechanism in skin. High temperature causes vasodilatation in skin arterioles and veins. At temperatures of 12–15°C, vasoconstriction of skin vessels occurs. This appears to be caused by noradrenergic stimulation of α_2-adrenoceptors. Below 12°C, paradoxical cold vasodilatation occurs. Neurotransmitter release is impaired. Vasodilator substances (e.g. prostaglandins) are released.

In most other tissues, vasodilatation occurs in response to cold. This is probably related to the predominance of α_1-receptors in other tissues compared with α_2-receptors in the skin.

Transmural pressure

This is the pressure across the wall of the vessel, and it can be affected by external and internal pressures:

- External pressure. Blood flow is impaired by a high external pressure outside the vessel (e.g. when muscle is contracted or when sitting or kneeling).
- Internal pressure. Initially, raised blood pressure causes the vessel to distend briefly. This causes the smooth muscle to be stretched, producing a contracting response. The vessel becomes constricted, increasing resistance and reducing flow within the vessel. This is termed the 'myogenic response', and it is a mechanism of autoregulation.

Distribution of cardiac output				
Organ	Mass (kg)	Blood flow (mL/min)	Blood flow per 100 g (mL/min/100 g)	Proportion of cardiac output (%)
Brain	1.4	750	54.0	13.9 [18.4]
Heart	0.3	250	84.0	4.7 [11.6]
Liver	1.5	1500*	100.0*	27.8 [20.4]*
(Gastrointestinal tract)	(2.5)	(1170)	(46.8)	(21.7 [16.0])
Kidneys	0.3	1260	420	23.3 [7.2]
Skeletal muscle	31.0	840	2.7	15.6 [20.0]
Skin	3.6	460	12.8	8.6 [4.8]
Rest of body	22.4	340	1.5	6.1 [17.6]
Whole body	63.0	5400	8.6	100 [100]

Fig. 4.1 Distribution of cardiac output to the various systems of the body. Note that the blood flow to the gastrointestinal tract (shown in round brackets) also flows through the liver via the portal circulation. Values for the liver marked * include the portal and arterial circulation to the liver. Values in square brackets denote the percentage of oxygen consumption by the various systems.

Local metabolites

Altered levels of many metabolites cause vasodilatation and increase perfusion of the tissue. These include:

- Hypoxia (i.e. decreased Po_2).
- Acidosis (caused by CO_2 and lactate).
- Adenosine triphosphate (ATP) breakdown products.
- K^+ (from contracting muscle and active brain neurons).
- Increase in osmolarity.

Different tissues are influenced to varying degrees by these factors; for example, coronary vessels react mainly to hypoxia and adenosine whereas cerebral vessels are influenced by K^+, H^+, and Pco_2.

Cytokines (previously known as autacoids)

Cytokines are chemical substances that are produced, secreted, and act locally as local hormones, producing local responses (e.g. inflammation, haemorrhage). They include:

- Histamine. This is an inflammatory mediator that causes arteriolar vasodilatation (H_1 receptor mediated). In veins, it causes vasoconstriction and increased permeability (H_2 receptor mediated).
- Bradykinin. This inflammatory mediator causes vasodilatation—nitric oxide (NO)-mediated—and increased vascular permeability (mediated by Ca^{2+}).
- 5-Hydroxytryptamine (5-HT, serotonin). This is found in platelets, the intestinal wall, and the central nervous system. It causes vasoconstriction. Production from platelets contributes significantly to vasoconstriction in response to vessel injury.
- Prostaglandins (PGs). These are inflammatory mediators synthesized from arachidonic acid by cyclooxygenase. They are produced by macrophages, leucocytes, fibroblasts, and endothelium. Their production is inhibited by non-steroidal anti-inflammatory drugs (NSAIDs) and steroids. PGF causes vasoconstriction, PGE causes vasodilatation, and PGI_2 (prostacyclin) causes vasodilatation.
- Thromboxane A_2. This is a platelet activator that causes vasoconstriction; it is involved in haemostasis.
- Leukotrienes. These are inflammatory mediators synthesized from arachidonic acid by lipoxygenase. They are produced by leucocytes, and they cause vasoconstriction and increased vascular permeability.
- Platelet activating factor (PAF). This is an inflammatory mediator that causes vasodilatation, increased vascular permeability, and vasospasm in hypoxic coronary vessels.

Endothelium-dependent relaxation and contraction

When stimulated, the endothelium of arteries and veins produce endothelium-derived relaxing factor (EDRF). EDRF was discovered to be nitric oxide (NO) and is produced in endothelial cells by cleavage from L-arginine by NO synthase. Stimuli include thrombin, bradykinin, substance-P, adenosine diphosphate (ADP), acetylcholine, and histamine.

NO diffuses into smooth muscle cells and activates an intracellular cyclic guanosine monophosphate (cGMP) messenger system, causing relaxation and vasodilatation.

The products of platelet activation stimulate NO release from intact endothelium to ensure that vasoconstriction only occurs with significant endothelial damage. Healthy endothelium will maintain vessel patency through NO, while injured endothelium will not counteract platelet-initiated vasoconstriction.

Blood flowing through an artery causes shear stress on the endothelial cell. When arterioles dilate to increase tissue perfusion, flow increases in feeder arteries by a process called flow-induced vasodilatation. This process is caused by increased shear stress, increasing NO production.

Vasoconstrictor substances are also produced by the endothelium—prostanoid is produced in large arteries to cause constriction in response to hypoxia; endothelin is a powerful vasoconstrictive peptide released in response to stretch, thrombin, and adrenaline. Endothelin acts locally, but it seems to have a role in the systemic regulation of blood pressure, and it has been the target for experimental therapeutic agents.

Autoregulation

Autoregulation is the process whereby tissue perfusion remains relatively constant even though blood pressure changes. It also keeps capillary filtration pressure at a stable value.

Flow is proportional to (pressure difference)/resistance. Therefore, to keep flow constant, any pressure change must be opposed by a resistance change. An increase in pressure causes arteriolar vasoconstriction, thereby increasing resistance. A decrease in pressure causes arteriolar vasodilatation and decreases resistance. It takes 30–60 s for the effect to take place so, for example, there is an initial increase in flow with a pressure increase before a steady state is reached.

Autoregulation only occurs over a limited pressure range. It is an intrinsic feature of the vessels, and it is independent of nervous control. However, it does not mean that tissue perfusion is constant all the time *in vivo*. Autoregulation can be reset to work at a new level by, for example, an increased sympathetic drive. The mechanisms for autoregulation are:

- Myogenic response. Increased pressure produces constriction of the vessel, opposing the rise in pressure and stabilizing blood flow.
- Vasodilator washout. This is the effect that blood flow has on the concentration of the local vasodilator metabolites. If blood flow increases, these metabolites are washed away faster, causing the vessel to constrict, thereby increasing resistance and slowing flow.
- In the heart, any increase in coronary arterial pressure causes a rise in tissue P_{O_2}, leading to vasoconstriction; this autoregulates heart blood flow.

Metabolic hyperaemia
Metabolic (or functional/active) hyperaemia is the increase in blood flow that occurs in exercising muscle and secreting exocrine glands when their metabolic rate increases. The production of local vasodilator metabolites leads to vasodilatation and causes vascular resistance to fall.

Flow-induced vasodilatation causes the main artery to dilate. Ascending dilatation from the arterioles to the feeder arteries leads to dilatation of the whole arterial tree supplying the tissue.

Blood flow in contracting muscle is increased in the resting phase. In the heart, the increase in metabolic rate causes a drop in tissue P_{O_2}, leading to vasodilatation.

Reactive hyperaemia
Reactive (or post-ischaemic) hyperaemia is the increase in blood flow that occurs after supply to a tissue has been temporarily interrupted.

Reactive hyperaemia enables resupply to ischaemic tissue as quickly as possible. The myogenic response is the predominant mechanism for brief occlusions, dilating the downstream vessels in preparation for the return of blood flow. In more prolonged occlusions, vasodilator metabolites

accumulate, and these play a significant role. Prostaglandins also aid this process.

Reactive hyperaemia is temporary, and it decays exponentially. A plateau of hyperaemia may precede decay in prolonged occlusions. In some tissues (e.g. the heart), there is oversupply of blood and oxygen compared with the deficit during the temporary interruption to flow.

Ischaemic reperfusion injury
When blood flow to a tissue is interrupted for a prolonged period reactive hyperaemia is impaired.

Reperfusion of ischaemic tissue results in superoxide ($O_2^{-\bullet}$) and hydroxide ($OH^\bullet$) radical formation. These damage the tissue and vessel wall, causing further occlusion. Damage is exacerbated by an increase in K^+ and tissue acidosis. Reperfused cells have an impaired plasmalemmal barrier to Ca^{2+} ions, which flow into the cell in an unrestricted way, causing calcium overload damage.

It is thought that reperfusion injury exacerbates damage to the myocardium, intestine and brain following ischaemia.

Most locally produced substances increase blood flow because the tissue wants to wash them away (e.g. lactate and adenosine are waste products of metabolism, which need to be removed).

Nervous control
Fig. 4.2 gives an overview of nervous control of the vasculature.

Sympathetic vasoconstrictor nerves
Sympathetic vasoconstrictor nerves innervate the vascular smooth muscle of the resistance and capacitance vessels. A basal level of activity of these nerves is responsible for vessel tone at rest. The neurotransmitter involved is noradrenaline, which acts on α_1-receptors on vascular smooth muscle causing contraction. When there is an increase in sympathetic drive:

- Vasoconstriction decreases local blood flow.
- Venoconstriction decreases local blood volume.
- Arteriolar constriction decreases capillary pressure, leading to greater resorption of

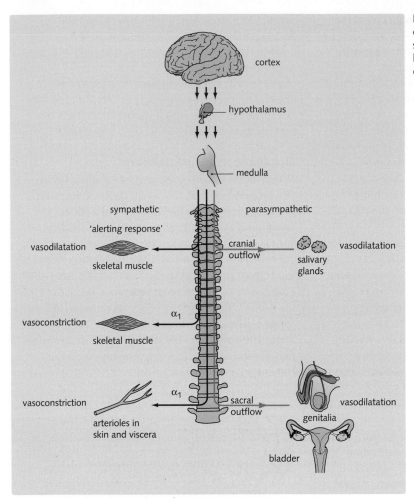

Fig. 4.2 Overview of nervous control of the vasculature. The sympathetic tracts are shown on the left and the parasympathetic tracts on the right.

fluid from the interstitium back into the blood.

If there is an increase in sympathetic activity throughout the body, total peripheral resistance and cardiac output increase. This constitutes the basis of the sympathetic response to haemorrhage.

A decrease in sympathetic activity causes vasodilatation and venodilatation.

Sympathetic vasodilator nerves

Some tissues (skeletal muscle and sweat glands) are also innervated by sympathetic vasodilator nerves. In skeletal muscle, vascular bed stimulation by these nerves (which use acetylcholine as the neurotransmitter and act on muscarinic receptors) causes vasodilatation. Stimulation only occurs as part of an 'alerting response', and it is initiated in the forebrain without any brainstem influence. The vasodilator effect is only temporary, and it plays no

role in blood pressure regulation. Stimulation of these nerves in sweat glands—probably involving vasoactive intestinal peptide (VIP) as neurotransmitter—produces sweating and cutaneous vasodilatation.

Parasympathetic vasodilator nerves

Parasympathetic vasodilator nerves innervate the blood vessels of:

- The head.
- Salivary glands.
- Pancreas.
- Gastrointestinal mucosa.
- Genitalia.
- Bladder.

The effect of these nerves on the total peripheral resistance is small because of their limited innervation. Their postganglionic neurons release acetylcholine, which relaxes vascular smooth muscle.

In some tissues (e.g. the pancreas), VIP may be the main neurotransmitter. Vasodilatation occurs in the arteries and arterioles of these vascular beds.

In the erectile tissue of the penis, it is parasympathetic and nitrergic vasodilatation that fills the corpus sinuses with blood, causing erection.

Nitrergic vasodilator nerves

Nitric oxide has recently been recognized as a neurotransmitter, both in the central and peripheral nervous system. Such neurons are referred to as nitrergic. They act on smooth muscle cells, causing relaxation. Nitrergic innervation has so far been found in the regulation of muscle tone in the gut and in sexual arousal in the male and female genitalia.

At present, pharmacological manipulation of nitrergic transmission is limited to the use of sildenafil (Viagra) in the treatment of male impotence. Sildenafil acts by selective inhibition of the phosphodiesterase present in smooth muscle of the genital vessels. This potentiates the effect of nitrergic stimulation (phosphodiesterase enzymes break up the cGMP that mediates the relaxation in response to NO). Sildenafil should not be given to hypotensive patients, nor combined with other forms of systemic nitrate treatment due to the risk of syncope.

Hormonal control

Although the vasculature is influenced by circulating hormones, short-term control is mainly achieved by the nervous system. Further details of these hormones can be found in *Crash Course: Endocrine and Reproductive Systems*.

Adrenaline

The catecholamines (adrenaline and noradrenaline) are secreted from the adrenal medulla.

More than three times as much adrenaline is secreted as noradrenaline. Plasma levels at rest of adrenaline are 0.1–0.5 nmol/L, and noradrenaline 0.5–3.0 nmol/L. There is more noradrenaline in plasma because of spill-over from sympathetic nerve terminals. Secretion is increased in exercise, hypotension, hypoglycaemia, and fight or flight situations.

Both hormones are β-adrenoceptor agonists, so they increase heart rate and contractility of the myocardium. Both hormones cause vasoconstriction in most tissues via α-receptors:

- Adrenaline causes vasoconstriction in most organs (especially skin), but vasodilatation in skeletal muscle, myocardium, and liver. This is because there are more β-receptors in these latter tissues, and adrenaline has a higher affinity for these receptors.
- Noradrenaline usually causes vasoconstriction because it has a higher affinity for α-receptors.

Adrenal gland stimulation results predominantly in adrenaline release. Effects on the heart include increased contractility, stroke volume, and heart rate. Blood pressure rises as a result, since the vasodilatory effects of adrenaline do not fully counteract the vasoconstrictor effects combined with the increased cardiac output.

Vasopressin (antidiuretic hormone)

Antidiuretic hormone (ADH) is a peptide produced in the hypothalamus and released from the posterior pituitary into the bloodstream. A rise in plasma osmolarity is the main stimulus for secretion. Falling blood pressure and volume are also stimuli, but to a lesser degree.

ADH promotes water retention by the kidney. High levels of ADH cause vasoconstriction in most tissues. In the brain and heart, NO-mediated vasodilatation occurs. This ensures preferential supply to the brain and heart in hypovolaemia.

Renin–angiotensin–aldosterone

Renin is an enzyme produced by the juxtaglomerular cells of the kidney. It converts angiotensinogen (from the liver) to angiotensin I (Fig. 4.3). Renin production is increased by:

- A fall in afferent arterial pressure to the glomeruli.
- Increased sympathetic activity.
- Decreased Na^+ in the macula densa of the adjacent tubule.

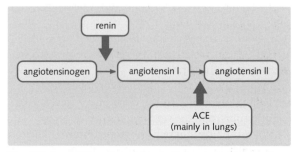

Fig. 4.3 Formation of angiotensin II. Angiotensinogen is secreted by the liver, acted on by renin (secreted by the kidney) and finally converted to the active angiotensin II by angiotensin-converting enzyme (ACE).

61

Angiotensin-converting enzyme (ACE) converts angiotensin I to the peptide angiotensin II (Fig. 4.3), which has the following actions:

- Increases aldosterone secretion from the adrenal cortex.
- Causes vasoconstriction at high concentration by acting directly on vascular smooth muscle, initiating release of noradrenaline from sympathetic nerve terminals, and increasing central sympathetic drive in the brainstem.
- Increases cardiac contractility.

Aldosterone increases salt and water retention by renal tubules.

Atrial natriuretic peptide

In response to high cardiac filling pressure, specialized myocytes in the atria secrete atrial natriuretic peptide (ANP). ANP increases the excretion of salt and water by renal tubules. It also has a small vasodilating effect.

Ventricles similarly secrete brain natriuretic peptide (BNP), which increases in heart failure. Levels of BNP may be used as a blood test for heart failure.

Cardiovascular receptors and central control

The cardiovascular system is ultimately regulated and controlled by the brain through autonomic nerves (Fig. 4.4).

Arterial baroreceptors and the baroreflex

Arterial baroreceptors (stretch receptors) are located in the carotid sinus and aortic arch. They play a key role in short-term blood pressure control, and they respond to stretch of the vessel wall. They continually produce impulses at normal vessel wall tone. Increased stretch (due to increased pressure) increases firing frequency, whereas decreased stretch decreases the firing rate.

The impulse that the baroreceptor generates is carried to the medulla by the glossopharyngeal nerves (carotid sinus) and the vagus nerves (aortic arch).

At the medulla, there is an interaction with the other central pathways. An increased firing rate causes the medulla to:

- Increase vagal (parasympathetic) drive.
- Decrease sympathetic drive.

This results in a decrease in heart rate. Contractility is probably not affected. It also causes a fall in total peripheral resistance. These measures all serve to reduce blood pressure back to normal. The baroreceptors are said to buffer the blood pressure in the short term.

When the baroreceptor is unloaded (stretch is reduced), the firing rate to the medulla is reduced. The effect is to decrease vagal and increase sympathetic drive. This results in:

- Increased heart rate and contractility.
- Peripheral vasoconstriction and venoconstriction.
- Catecholamine secretion.
- Increased renin secretion.

The effect is to increase cardiac output, total peripheral resistance, and the circulating volume, all of which serve to return blood pressure to normal.

The baroreflex is very rapid (<1 s for bradycardia to occur), and it is very important in acute hypotension and haemorrhage.

The sensitivity of the arterial baroreceptors to a change in blood pressure is decreased by:

- Age. The compliance of the arterial wall falls with age, which means there is less stretch of the arterial walls.
- Chronic hypertension. The arterial wall loses its distensibility.

The baroreflex is inhibited by stimulation of the hypothalamic defence area in fight or flight situations.

The level of blood pressure that the baroreceptor takes as normal (the setting or set point) can be reset by central or peripheral processes:

- Central resetting. In exercise, the rise in blood pressure that occurs does not cause a bradycardia because there has been a central influence to operate the baroreflex at a new higher level. The neurons that drive inspiration inhibit cardiac vagal nerves, so blocking baroreceptor impulses and causing a decreased vagal drive. This explains the increased heart rate with inspiration (sinus arrhythmia).
- Peripheral resetting. Chronic hyper- or hypotension leads to the set point being reset to this new pressure. This allows the baroreflex to operate in its optimal range. This is also the reason why the baroreflex is not very useful for long-term blood pressure homeostasis.

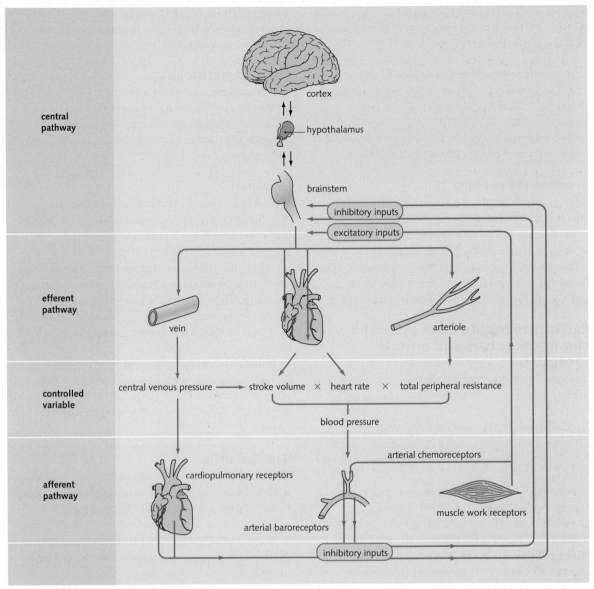

Fig. 4.4 Overview of the central control of the circulation. (Adapted from Levick R. *Introducing Cardiovascular Physiology*. Butterworth–Heinemann, 1995. Reproduced by permission of Edward Arnold Ltd.)

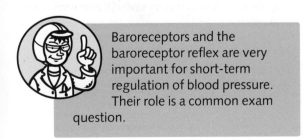

Baroreceptors and the baroreceptor reflex are very important for short-term regulation of blood pressure. Their role is a common exam question.

Cardiopulmonary receptors

There are many cardiopulmonary receptors connected to afferent fibres innervating the heart, great veins, and pulmonary artery. Overall, stimulation of these receptors causes bradycardia, vasodilatation, and hypotension. There are three main classes of receptor with differing functions— venoatrial stretch receptors, unmyelinated mechanoreceptor fibres, and chemosensitive fibres.

Venoatrial stretch receptors

These are branched nerve endings located where the great veins join the atria. They are connected to large myelinated vagal fibres. Stimulation produces a reflex tachycardia by selectively increasing sympathetic drive to the pacemaker. There is also an increase in salt and water excretion.

Unmyelinated mechanoreceptor fibres
These are present in both atria and in the left ventricle. Afferent fibres travel in vagal and sympathetic nerves. Large distension stimulates these receptors, causing an inhibitory effect. Reflex bradycardia and peripheral vasodilatation occurs.

Chemosensitive fibres
Some unmyelinated vagal and sympathetic afferents are chemosensitive. They are stimulated in response to bradykinin and other substances released by an ischaemic myocardium. It is thought that the pain of angina and myocardial infarction are caused by these fibres. Stimulation increases respiration as well as causing bradycardia and peripheral vasodilatation.

Excitatory inputs from arterial chemoreceptors and muscle receptors
Chemoreceptors are located in the carotid and aortic bodies. They are nerve terminals whose excitation is increased by hypoxia, hypercapnia, and acidosis of arterial blood (see *Crash Course: Respiratory System*). Their fibres travel with afferent baroreceptor fibres in the glossopharyngeal and vagus nerves.

At normal gas tensions, chemoreceptors are mainly involved in the control of breathing. However, when their excitation is increased, they respond by causing a sympathetically mediated vasoconstriction and a mild bradycardia. The respiratory chemoreflex increases tidal volume, which stimulates lung stretch receptors. This causes a marked tachycardia and a modest vasodilatation. Overall, the heart rate and blood pressure increase to enhance perfusion. The chemoreflex plays an important role in asphyxia, severe haemorrhage, and hypotension, where the chemoreceptors are excited by the reduced metabolite supply (and blood pressure is below baroreceptor range).

Skeletal muscle produces a reflex cardiovascular response to exercise. This is stimulated by metaboloreceptors (activated by K^+ and H^+) and mechanoreceptors (activated by pressure and tension). The excitation travels through small nerve fibres (groups III and IV). The reflex produces tachycardia, increased myocardial contractility, and vasoconstriction in other vascular beds. This allows greater perfusion of the exercising muscle. This is termed the exercise pressor response, and it is greater in static exercise.

Central pathways
The central pathways that influence the cardiovascular system have only been partly explained. They involve a complex interaction between the medulla, hypothalamus, cerebellum, and cortex.

Medulla
It used to be thought that there was a specific vasomotor centre in the medulla. Now, it is thought that there are complex signals between the hypothalamus, cortex, and cerebellum as well as signals within the vasomotor centre of the medulla. The rostral ventrolateral medulla is responsible for the sympathetic outflow, whereas the nucleus ambiguous is responsible for the parasympathetic outflow; these two areas control vessel tone and heart rate.

Information from baroreceptors is received (at the nucleus tractus solitarius) by the medulla, and it is relayed to the hypothalamus. Medullary autonomic control is also influenced by hypothalamic activity.

Hypothalamus
This contains four areas of interest:
- Depressor area. This can produce the baroreflex, but it is not vital for the reflex to occur.
- Defence area. This is responsible for the alerting response and the fight or flight response. It, therefore, plays a role in governing sympathetic outflow.
- Temperature-regulating area. This controls cutaneous vascular tone and sweating.
- Vasopressin-secreting area. This produces vasopressin, which travels through nerve axons to the pituitary.

Cerebellum
The cerebellum's primary role is muscle coordination. During exercise, the cerebellum helps to coordinate the response to exercise.

Cortex
The cortex may initiate many of the cardiovascular responses. The effects of fear and emotion on the vasculature probably have a cortical influence.

Regulation of circulation in individual tissues

Blood flow rates in various circulations are given in Fig. 4.5.

Coronary circulation

Myocardial oxygen demand is very high, being about 8 mL O_2/min/100 g. During exercise, cardiac work can increase five-fold, thereby increasing oxygen demand. Oxygen levels in coronary venous blood are very low, so demand can only be met by increasing flow.

Oxygen transport is aided by the high capillary density (large area and decreased distance for exchange) and the presence of myoglobin. There is a high oxygen extraction from the capillaries (>60%) even at rest.

Blood flow is mainly controlled by tissue P_{O_2}. Low P_{O_2} produces a metabolic hyperaemia. Metabolic vasodilatation can be partly opposed by sympathetic α_1-noradrenergic vasoconstriction. Adrenaline acts on β_2-receptors in coronary smooth muscle to dilate the vessels.

Coronary arteries are functional end-arteries with few cross-connections between them. They are at risk of being blocked by thrombosis, causing ischaemia. There are, however, some collateral vessels, which may delay the onset of ischaemia.

Flow rate in various circulations		
Circulation	Basal flow rate (mL/min/100 g)	Maximum flow rate (minimum) (mL/min/100 g)
Coronary	80	400
Phasic (white, fast) skeletal muscle	3	200 (on exercise)
Tonic (red, slow) skeletal muscle	15	200 (on exercise)
Cutaneous	10–20 (at 27°C)	200
Brain Grey matter	55 100	—
Renal	400	—
Liver GIT	85 40	150 (after food) 80 (after food)

Fig. 4.5 Resting and maximum blood flow rates in the various circulations. (GIT, gastrointestinal tract.)

During systole, coronary artery branches in the myocardium are compressed. Flow is fully restored only during diastole (Fig. 4.6).

Skeletal muscle

Oxygen and nutrient delivery to the muscle cells must increase with exercise. Removal of waste products and heat must also be increased during exercise.

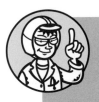

Skeletal muscle makes up 40% of body mass. Its vasculature contributes significantly to vascular resistance and, therefore, affects blood pressure homeostasis.

Phasically active muscle consists of white fibres (e.g. gastrocnemius). Postural muscles (e.g. soleus) are tonically active red fibres, and they have a greater capillary density.

Sympathetic vasoconstrictor nerve reflexes controlled by baroreceptors play a major role in controlling flow. In hypovolaemia, for example, vasoconstriction can reduce flow in skeletal muscle to one fifth of its resting value.

During exercise, metabolic vasodilatation is the dominant mechanism for increasing flow. Adrenaline causes vasodilatation by acting on smooth-muscle β_2-receptors.

At rest, only 25% of the oxygen in the blood is extracted. In severe exercise, this extraction can be increased considerably. Extraction is aided by the presence of myoglobin.

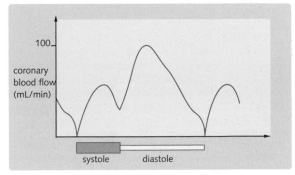

Fig. 4.6 Coronary blood flow during the cardiac cycle. Note that maximal blood flow is during diastole.

The skeletal muscle pump aids venous return to the heart. This lowers venous pressure in the limbs. The pressure difference from the arterial to venous circulations increases. Thus, the perfusion pressure is increased, driving blood flow.

Blood flow is impaired during contraction. If contraction is sustained then the fibres will become hypoxic. Lactate will accumulate causing pain, and strength will be rapidly lost.

An increase in the capillary filtration rate can lead to a fall in plasma volume.

Cutaneous circulation

The skin has a low metabolic requirement, and its vasculature is mainly involved in the regulation of the internal core body temperature.

Specific areas of the skin have arteriovenous anastomoses (Fig. 4.7). These exposed areas have a high surface area to volume ratio and include the fingers, toes, palms, soles of the feet, lips, nose, and ears. These anastomoses are controlled by sympathetic vasoconstrictor nerves. In turn the sympathetic activity is controlled via the brainstem by the temperature-regulating area in the hypothalamus. The nerves controlling sweating are also controlled in the same way—when the core body temperature is too high, sympathetic drive is reduced and the arteriovenous anastomoses dilate.

Skin temperature is very variable as it is influenced by ambient temperature. It has a direct effect on cutaneous vascular tone:

- Local heating causes vasodilatation.
- Local cooling causes vasoconstriction.

Paradoxical cold vasodilatation occurs in acral areas (the extremities) on prolonged exposure to cold.

After the initial vasoconstriction, vasodilatation occurs. This is thought to be because the cold impairs sympathetic vasoconstriction. This phenomenon prevents skin damage in such exposure.

Skin temperature receptors can evoke a weak spinal reflex that changes sympathetic vasomotor activity.

Hypotension causes a neural and hormonal (angiotensin, ADH, and adrenaline) vasoconstriction of skin vessels. This produces the cold skin seen in shock.

Exercise causes vasoconstriction of the skin initially, but this can become a dilatation if the core temperature rises.

Emotion can produce a hyperaemic response in the skin (blushing) and the gastric and colonic mucosa.

Compression of the skin for long periods (e.g. when sitting) impairs blood flow. Reactive hyperaemia and the skin's high tolerance to hypoxia prevents ischaemic damage. Restlessness (i.e. the desire to move position) also plays a major role, possibly stimulated by local metabolites and pain receptors. In certain patients, however, failure to move or be moved can lead to necrosis in compressed areas (bed sores).

In hot weather, cutaneous vasodilatation can lower central venous pressure. This can lead to fainting (e.g. the soldier while standing to attention on a hot day must use his skeletal muscle pump to maintain venous pressure, otherwise he will suddenly faint).

Cerebral circulation

Grey matter has a high oxygen consumption (7 mL O_2/min/100 g). As grey matter has little tolerance to hypoxia, consciousness is lost after a few seconds of ischaemia.

The main task of the entire cardiovascular system is to maintain an adequate supply of oxygen to the brain. The cerebral circulation can adjust itself locally to meet local demand. This is mainly by an increase in interstitial K^+, causing metabolic hyperaemia.

In young people, the circle of Willis enables blood supply to be maintained if one carotid artery is occluded. These anastomoses linking the supply arteries together are less effective in the elderly. There is a high capillary density, similar in size to that in the myocardium. The presence of a blood–brain barrier tightly controls the neuronal environment. Lipid-soluble molecules can diffuse freely, but ionic solutes cannot.

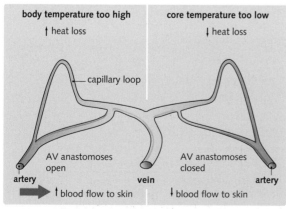

Fig. 4.7 Temperature control by arteriovenous (AV) anastomoses.

The brain can control cardiac output and vascular resistance of other tissues through autonomic nerves. Cerebral perfusion is maintained at the expense of other tissues when required.

There is good autoregulation of the cerebral blood flow, but this fails when pressure falls below 50 mmHg.

Cerebral vessels are very sensitive to arterial P_{CO_2}:
- Hypercapnia causes vasodilatation (Fig. 4.8).
- Hypocapnia causes vasoconstriction.

Reduction in arterial P_{CO_2} through hyperventilation can lead to cerebral vasoconstriction, and even transient unconsciousness. Cerebral vessels do not participate in baroreflex vasoconstriction.

Pulmonary circulation

The entire output of the right ventricle enters the pulmonary circulation. A separate bronchial circulation from the aorta meets the metabolic needs of the bronchi.

There is a very high capillary density and very thin blood–alveolar surface to maximize gaseous exchange. Gas exchange in the lung is flow limited (i.e. a rise in blood flow increases the rate of oxygen uptake).

Pulmonary arteries and arterioles are shorter, thinner walled, and more easily distensible than systemic vessels so that pulmonary vascular resistance is very low with a low pulmonary arterial pressure (22/8 mmHg). There is no autoregulation of blood flow, although the pulmonary vessels still respond to systemic mediators (e.g. adrenaline).

Low capillary pressure means that there is no filtration of fluid into the alveoli in health.

In the upright person, mean arterial pressure at the apex of the lung is about 3 mmHg and at the base is about 21 mmHg. At the level of the heart, the mean pressure is 15 mmHg. At the lung base, high pressure causes the thin-walled vessels to distend and blood flow to increase (Fig. 4.8). At the apex, flow only occurs during systole, as the diastolic pressure is insufficient to open the vessels.

The ventilation–perfusion ratio governs the efficiency of oxygen transfer. Although ventilation is greater at the base than at the apex, the difference is not as great as the difference in flow. This implies that ventilation–perfusion ratio is higher at the apex than at the base, and this mismatch impairs efficiency.

General hypoxia causes pulmonary hypertension. Poorly ventilated areas become poorly perfused because of hypoxic vasoconstriction. This mechanism helps to optimize ventilation–perfusion ratios.

Renal circulation

Renal blood flow is autoregulated over a certain range of blood pressure. This allows a near-constant glomerular filtration rate. Autoregulation fails in severe hypotension (prerenal failure).

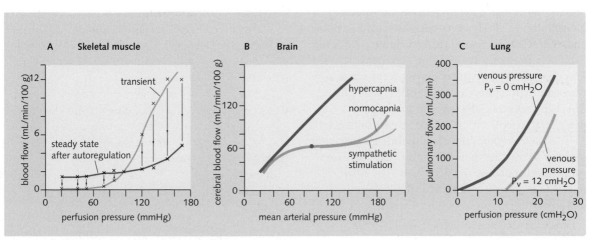

Fig. 4.8 Pressure–flow curves for (A) skeletal muscle, (B) brain vasculature, and (C) lung tissue. In (A) one line shows transient flow after altering perfusion pressure; the other line shows steady state achieved by autoregulation. (B) shows autoregulation at normal arterial P_{CO_2} and the effect of hypercapnia. In (C) the airway pressure was constant at 4 cmH$_2$O. Increasing perfusion pressure increases pulmonary flow due to vascular distension and opening of some closed venous vessels. This increase in flow is less marked when venous pressure is above airway pressure.

the body is very good at diverting blood flow to where it is needed. However, some circulations (e.g. cerebral and renal) are special in that their blood flow is usually preserved at the expense of others.

Mesenteric circulation

The hyperaemia associated with the arrival of food is caused by:

- Local hormones (e.g. gastrin and cholecystokinin).
- Digestion products (e.g. glucose and fatty acids).
- Increased vagal activity.

The rise in mesenteric/splanchnic blood flow produces a tachycardia and, therefore, an increase in cardiac output of 1 L/min. There is also vasoconstriction in skeletal muscle vascular beds. There is normally no significant change in blood pressure.

Coordinated cardiovascular responses

Cardiovascular response to posture

When moving from supine to standing (orthostasis), the effect of gravity on venous blood causes venous pooling in the legs. There is a fall in intrathoracic blood volume. This leads to decreased cardiac filling and, therefore, decreased stroke volume. This leads to a fall in pressure. This is often corrected immediately by the baroreflex, but it can cause a transient hypotension, even in healthy individuals. This happens especially when there is already peripheral vasodilatation in a warm environment.

The baroreceptors and cardiopulmonary receptors react by decreasing their firing rate. This increases sympathetic outflow and decreases vagal drive, resulting in an increased heart rate (of about 20 beats/min) and contractility. Peripheral vasoconstriction increases total peripheral resistance, which helps increase blood pressure. Venoconstriction also plays a limited role in helping to reverse venous pooling. Capillary filtration in the leg increases because of the increase in venous pressure. This may cause a drop in plasma volume

over time. Vasopressin and aldosterone (via renin–angiotensin) reduce salt and water excretion in order to increase plasma volume. The overall effect is a maintenance of arterial pressure and, thus, cerebral perfusion.

Failure of this mechanism causes postural hypotension (i.e. fainting on standing). Always record blood pressure lying and standing.

Valsalva manoeuvre

This is a forced expiration against a closed glottis. This commonly occurs when coughing, defecating, and lifting heavy weights. It produces a raised intrathoracic pressure (Fig. 4.9).

This manoeuvre is a useful test of baroreceptor competence. If the pressure fall in phase 2 continues and there is no bradycardia in phase 4, then the baroreflex is being interrupted, leading to postural hypotension.

Cardiovascular response to exercise

Initial requirements during exercise are:

- Increased gaseous exchange in the pulmonary circulation.
- Increased blood flow to the working muscle.
- Stable blood pressure.

Cardiac output and oxygen uptake

Cardiac output is increased by increases in heart rate or stroke volume (Fig. 4.10):

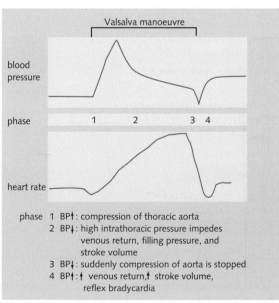

Fig. 4.9 Response to the Valsalva manoeuvre. (BP, blood pressure.)

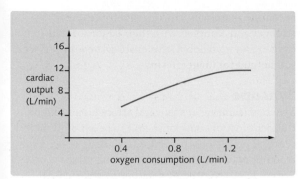

Fig. 4.10 Relationship between cardiac output and oxygen consumption in the whole body. It shows a linear increase of cardiac output with oxygen consumption produced by increased heart rate and stroke volume.

- Increased heart rate can be caused by sympathetic stimulation or decreased vagal inhibition.
- Stroke volume can be increased by increased cardiac filling (due to skeletal muscle pump and splanchnic vasoconstriction), increased contractility (due to sympathetic stimulation), or a fall in peripheral resistance (due to skeletal muscle vasodilatation).

In upright exercise, stroke volume plays the main role in increasing output. In supine exercise, heart rate increases mainly account for the increased output. Stroke volume increases only at low work rates.

Changes in blood flow to active muscle

Blood flow to active muscle increases with exercise. Hyperaemia can be as much as 40 times normal flow, and it is caused by:
- Metabolic vasodilatation.
- Increased pressure gradient by skeletal muscle pump in upright exercise.
- Capillary recruitment by dilatation of terminal arterioles.

The alerting response caused by anticipation of exercise (e.g. at the start of a race) causes an initial sympathetically mediated vasodilatation.

Changes in blood flow in other tissues

Coronary blood flow increases with the increase in cardiac work. Cutaneous vessels initially contract to maintain blood pressure, but dilate if core temperature rises. Vasoconstriction in the renal, splanchnic, and non-active muscle vascular beds helps to maintain blood pressure.

Blood pressure during static and dynamic exercise

In dynamic (alternately contracting and relaxing) exercise, the diastolic pressure hardly changes although the pulse pressure rises (Fig. 4.11). The increase in pressure in static exercise is caused by the exercise pressor response, which is mediated by receptors in the muscle (see p. 64).

Initiation of the response to exercise

The exact causes of the changes in autonomic activity during exercise are not known. Two hypotheses are prevalent:
- The central command hypothesis. This postulates that as the cerebral cortex initiates contraction of muscle, it also instructs the autonomic nerves of the brainstem to increase heart rate. Baroreflex resetting to a higher value may also be linked to this theory.
- The peripheral reflex hypothesis. The nerve receptors in working muscle are excited by the presence of chemical stimulants, and they cause a reflex sympathetic response, increasing cardiac output and pressure.

It is likely that the central command hypothesis produces the initial tachycardia and vagal suppression. The peripheral reflex hypothesis

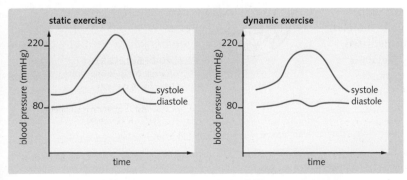

Fig. 4.11 Blood pressure during static and dynamic exercise. Diastolic pressure rises in static exercise, but it remains relatively constant in dynamic exercise. The cardiac work is greater for equivalent static than for dynamic exercise.

probably accounts for the slower increase in cardiac output and peripheral vasoconstriction.

Cardiovascular response to training

This is most important in the long-distance or endurance athlete. Training causes improvements in oxygen transport rate and changes in cardiac structure and function. Causes of improved oxygen delivery and extraction are:

- New capillaries formed in skeletal muscle.
- More muscle mitochondria closer to capillaries.
- Increased muscle myoglobin concentration.

Changes in cardiac structure and function are:

- Thicker ventricular wall.
- Increased myocardial vascularity.
- Increased ventricular cavity size.

Stroke volume is much higher because of the cardiac changes. Most athletes have a resting bradycardia, but because of the increased stroke volume the resting cardiac output is the same.

In exercise, the athlete's maximum heart rate is the same as that for an untrained subject, but because the athlete starts at a lower value, a much greater change can be achieved. This, coupled with the increased stroke volume, means that the athlete can increase cardiac output up to as much as 35 L/min.

Diving reflex

The diving reflex occurs when cold water touches the facial receptors of the trigeminal nerve. The body is expecting a dive into water and a period of submersion. The limited oxygen must be preferentially diverted to the heart and brain. There are three reflexes involved:

- Apnoea—Arterial chemoreceptors are triggered as asphyxia develops.
- Bradycardia—caused by intense vagal inhibition of the pacemaker.
- Peripheral vasoconstriction—occurs in the splanchnic, renal, and skeletal muscle vascular beds. The strong, sympathetically mediated vasoconstriction overwhelms any metabolic dilatation that may occur in active muscle.

In marine mammals, the diving reflex is much stronger and, coupled with their larger store of oxygen and myoglobin, this enables them to survive submerged for longer periods.

Syncope

Syncope (fainting or vasovagal attack) is a sudden, transient loss of consciousness as a result of impaired cerebral perfusion. It is caused by a drop in cerebral blood flow to less than half its normal value.

It may be initiated by a pathophysiological cause (e.g. orthostasis or severe hypovolaemia) or by psychological stress (e.g. fear, pain, or horror). In psychogenic fainting, there is often a pre-faint period of tachycardia, cutaneous vasoconstriction, hyperventilation, and sweating. A vasovagal faint proceeds as follows:

1. A sudden increase in vagal inhibition leads to bradycardia.
2. Peripheral vasodilatation results due to decreased sympathetic drive.
3. This causes a fall in blood pressure, reducing cerebral blood flow.
4. Loss of consciousness results within seconds.

The cause of the sudden changes is unknown. In psychogenic fainting, it could be a primitive 'playing dead' response. In hypovolaemic fainting, it could be triggered by mechanoreceptors in the near-empty left ventricle.

The person who has fainted ends up in the supine position. This raises the intrathoracic blood volume and the filling pressure. Coupled with the baroreflex, this then increases cardiac output and arterial pressure. Consciousness is restored in about two minutes.

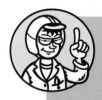

To understand the cardiovascular responses, first decide what has changed and then think how the body might restore the status quo.

- List the mechanisms involved in the local control of blood flow.
- Explain how nitric oxide is involved in regulating blood flow and vessel diameter.
- How is autoregulation brought about and what is its importance?
- What is the role of the sympathetic vasoconstrictor nerves in vascular control?
- Explain how and where vasodilator nerves (sympathetic and parasympathetic) operate.
- What are the principal vasoactive hormones? How do they affect the vasculature?
- What is the baroreflex? How is it elicited?
- What are the roles of venoatrial stretch receptors and mechanoreceptors?
- What effects do the chemosensitive receptors have on the cardiovascular system?
- What areas of the brain influence central control?
- With regard to the specialized regulation of the vascular system in different organs:
  - What is the average resting flow in each organ?
  - How does the regulation of flow within that organ relate to its function?
  - Explain how each organ responds to its special circumstances.
- How does orthostasis affect cardiac output? What are the reflexes involved in maintaining blood pressure?
- How does the Valsalva manoeuvre affect the heart and blood pressure? What can it tell us?
- Describe the changes that occur in exercise. How are they brought about?
- Explain how and why there are differences in the response to static and dynamic exercise.
- How does the physiology of a top athlete differ from that of the general populace?
- Describe the diving reflex.
- Why does fainting occur? What receptors and reflexes are involved in the different causes?

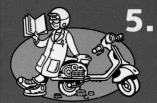

5. The Cardiovascular System in Disease

Shock and haemorrhage

Shock

Definition
Shock is an acute failure of the cardiovascular system to adequately perfuse the tissues of the body.

There are four major shock categories depending upon the causative factor:
- Hypovolaemic shock.
- Septicaemic shock.
- Cardiogenic shock.
- Anaphylactic shock.

Symptoms
The symptoms of shock are:
- Faintness, light-headedness, dizziness.
- Sweating.
- Reduced level of consciousness.

Signs
The classical signs of shock are:
- Pale, cold, clammy skin caused by cutaneous vasoconstriction in an effort to conserve blood flow to the vital organs and sweating caused by sympathetic stimulation.
- Rapid, weak pulse caused by tachycardia and decreased stroke volume.
- Reduced pulse pressure.
- Rapid, shallow breathing.
- Impaired renal output.
- Muscular weakness.
- Confusion or reduced awareness.

Hypovolaemic shock
This results from a fall in circulating blood volume caused by either:
- External fluid loss (e.g. vomiting, diarrhoea, haemorrhage).
- Internal fluid loss (e.g. pancreatitis, severe burns, internal bleeding).

Septicaemic shock
Septicaemic shock is caused by toxins (e.g. endotoxin) released from bacteria during infection. The patient may have warm skin, but will have a low blood pressure due to inappropriate vasodilatation.

Treatment can include adrenaline and vasoconstrictors. Artificial ventilation is sometimes required for lung involvement if respiratory distress syndrome develops.

Cardiogenic shock
This is caused by an interruption of cardiac function such that the heart is unable to maintain the circulation. It usually has an acute onset, but it may be a result of worsening heart failure. Causes include:
- Myocardial infarction.
- Arrhythmia.
- Cardiac tamponade.
- Myocarditis.
- Infective endocarditis.
- Pulmonary embolus.
- Tension pneumothorax.
- Aortic dissection.

Cardiogenic shock should not be treated with adrenaline under any circumstances as this will exacerbate the cardiac problem.

Anaphylactic shock
This is a type I hypersensitivity reaction, which is an immediate IgE-mediated immune response to an antigen in the body to which the patient is allergic. It leads to circulatory collapse, dyspnoea, and even death.

The IgE immune response consists of the activation of basophils and mast cells (basophils are mobile in the blood, mast cells are fixed in tissue). The degranulation of these cells leads to release of histamine and other factors. Prostaglandins, leukotrienes, thromboxane, and platelet activation factors are also synthesized and released. The results are as follows:
- Generalized peripheral vasodilatation, which leads to hypotension.
- Increased vascular permeability reducing plasma volume.
- Bronchial smooth muscle constriction, which leads to dyspnoea.
- Oral, laryngeal, and pharyngeal oedema.
- Urticaria and flushing.

Death may result from the circulatory collapse.

Treatment consists of immediate intramuscular adrenaline and infusion of hydrocortisone (a glucocorticoid).

An anaphylactoid reaction produces a similar picture to that described above, but it is caused by the direct effects of a substance on mast cells and basophils (i.e. it is not mediated by IgE). This sometimes occurs with radio-opaque contrast media.

Cardiovascular responses to blood loss

A 10% blood loss produces little change in blood pressure. A 20–30% blood loss causes shock, but it is not usually life threatening. A 30–40% blood loss produces severe or irreversible shock (50–70 mmHg fall in blood pressure). Hypotension is an indirect result of blood loss. It is caused by a decreased blood volume, reducing venous return to the heart. A reduced end-diastolic volume reduces the strength of contraction and, therefore, stroke volume.

The body responds in different ways to rectify the loss of pressure and volume. The response is often subdivided into:

- An immediate response occurring within seconds (Fig. 5.1).
- An intermediate response occurring within minutes or hours (Fig. 5.2).
- A long-term response occurring within days or weeks (Fig. 5.3).

Treatment is to prevent further blood loss and volume expansion with intravenous fluids.

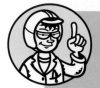 In haemorrhage, the body loses blood. It must attempt to maintain vital perfusion and blood pressure. Then, it will try to rectify the loss. The receptors, reflexes, and responses reflect this aim.

Hypertension

Current World Health Organization (WHO) recommendations define hypertension as a resting blood pressure above 140 mmHg systolic and/or 90 mmHg diastolic in those under 50 years, and 160 mmHg systolic and/or 95 mmHg diastolic in older patients, although these criteria are somewhat arbitrary. Cardiovascular disease risks increase with blood pressure even within the normal range. Using the WHO criteria, up to 25% of the population may have hypertension.

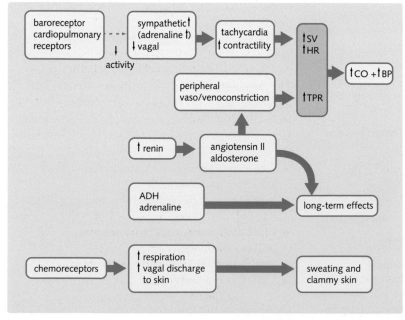

Fig. 5.1 Immediate response to haemorrhage. (ADH, antidiuretic hormone; BP, blood pressure; CO, cardiac output; HR, heart rate; SV, stroke volume; TPR, total peripheral resistance.)

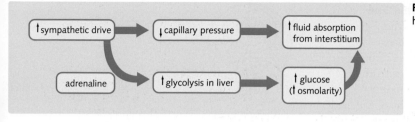

Fig. 5.2 Intermediate response to haemorrhage.

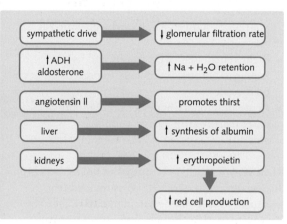

Fig. 5.3 Long-term response to haemorrhage. (ADH, antidiuretic hormone.)

Classification

Hypertension is classified according to both underlying cause and clinical progression. Primary (essential) hypertension accounts for 90% of hypertensive patients; the precise aetiology is unknown, but it is probably multifactorial. Predisposing factors include:

- Age (blood pressure rises with age).
- Obesity.
- Excessive alcohol intake.
- High salt intake.
- Genetic susceptibility.

Smoking increases cardiovascular risk in hypertensive patients.

Secondary hypertension accounts for the remaining 10% of cases. Here, the hypertension arises as a result of other disease processes:

- Renal disease—chronic glomerulonephritis, chronic pyelonephritis, polycystic renal disease, renal artery stenosis.
- Endocrine disease—Cushing's syndrome, Conn's syndrome, adrenal hyperplasia, phaeochromocytoma, acromegaly, corticosteroid therapy.
- Congenital disease—coarctation of the aorta.

- Neurological disease—raised intracranial pressure, brainstem lesions.
- Pregnancy—pre-eclampsia.

The clinical progression of hypertension can be classified as benign or malignant. Benign hypertension is a stable elevation of blood pressure over a period of many years (usually recognized in patients aged over 40 years). Malignant (accelerated) hypertension is an acute, severe elevation of blood pressure.

Complications

Hypertension is a major risk factor for:

- Atherosclerosis.
- Intracerebral haemorrhage—also known as cerebrovascular accident (CVA).
- Aortic aneurysm.
- Cardiac failure (which is the cause of death in one third of patients).
- Visual disturbance (caused by papilloedema and retinal haemorrhages).

Note that initially hypertension is usually asymptomatic, and in essential hypertension no obvious cause can be found. This can affect compliance with therapy, especially if drugs have too many side effects.

The distinction between primary and secondary hypertension is of great clinical significance, since only in the latter case is treatment of the underlying cause possible.

Hypertensive vascular disease

Hypertension not only accelerates atherosclerosis, but it also results in characteristic changes to arterioles and small arteries. All these changes are associated with narrowing of the vessel lumen. Changes in benign hypertension include:

- In arteries—muscular hypertrophy of the media, reduplication of the external lamina, and intimal thickening.
- In arterioles—hyaline arteriosclerosis (protein deposits in wall).
- In vessels of the brain—microaneurysms (Charcot–Bouchard aneurysms) can occur.

Other changes are associated with, but not restricted to, malignant hypertension. Hyperplastic arteriosclerosis, with reduplication of basement membrane and muscular hypertrophy solely within the intima can occur in arteries and arterioles.

When these changes are associated with fibrin deposition (also known as fibrinoid changes) and necrosis of the vessel wall, the condition is known as necrotizing arteriolitis. These changes frequently affect the renal arterioles to produce nephrosclerosis, which may impair renal function or exacerbate hypertension through the renin–angiotensin system.

Hypertensive heart disease
Systemic (left-sided) hypertensive heart disease

Criteria for diagnosis of systemic hypertensive heart disease are:

- History of hypertension (>140/90 mmHg).
- Left ventricular hypertrophy (wall thickness measuring >15 mm, weighing >500 g).
- Absence of any other causes of hypertrophy.

In hypertensive heart disease, changes that are initially adaptive lead to cardiac dilatation, congestive heart failure, and even sudden death. The heart adapts with hypertrophy of the left ventricular wall, initially without any change in ventricular volume. Histologically this is characterized by enlargement of the myocytes and their nuclei (hypertrophy). In the long term, interstitial fibrosis and myocyte atrophy occur, causing ventricular dilatation.

Pulmonary hypertensive heart disease (cor pulmonale)

Pulmonary hypertensive heart disease can be defined as right ventricular hypertrophy (wall thickness measuring >10 mm) as a result of

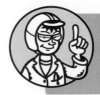

When trying to remember that benign hypertension causes hyaline changes to arterioles think be-nine and hya-line.

hypertension in the pulmonary circulation caused by lung disorder.

Pulmonary hypertension can be classified as either:

- Right ventricular hypertrophy and failure (also known as chronic pulmonary hypertension or cor pulmonale).
- Acute pulmonary hypertension (a sudden onset usually after a large pulmonary emboli).

Right ventricular hypertrophy and failure is a chronic disease of right ventricular pressure load (e.g. pulmonary vasoconstriction in hypoxia caused by high altitude or in chronic obstructive airways disease). Right ventricular dilatation may cause tricuspid regurgitation.

Pulmonary artery hypertension may be caused by heart disease (left ventricular failure, mitral valve disease, cardiac shunts) or lung disease (primary pulmonary hypertension, interstitial fibrosis, pulmonary emboli).

Antihypertensive drugs
Angiotensin-converting enzyme inhibitors

Angiotensin-converting enzyme (ACE) inhibitors (e.g. captopril, enalapril, perindopril) inhibit the conversion of angiotensin I to angiotensin II by ACE (Fig. 5.4). They also inhibit bradykinin (a vasodilator) breakdown by ACE. They are now becoming a first-line treatment, but they should not be used to treat patients with severe renal artery stenosis.

The side effects are:
- First-dose hypotension.
- Skin rash.
- Coughing.
- Renal impairment.

Perindopril is a once-a-day preparation with a lower incidence of first-dose hypotension.

Risks can be further minimized if the patient takes a once daily preparation at night when he or she is lying down.

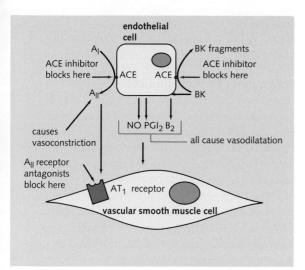

Fig. 5.4 Action of angiotensin-converting enzyme (ACE) inhibitors and angiotensin II (A$_{II}$) receptor antagonists. (A$_I$, angiotensin I; A$_{II}$, angiotensin II; AT$_1$, angiotensin II receptor type 1; B$_2$, activated bradykinin—activated by endothelial cell; BK, bradykinin; NO, nitric oxide; PGI$_2$, prostacyclin.)

Angiotensin II receptor antagonists

Angiotensin II receptor antagonists (e.g. losartan) inhibit the angiotensin II receptor and prevent the action of angiotensin II (see Fig. 5.4). Unlike the ACE inhibitors, they do not affect bradykinin. They are useful when ACE inhibitors have produced an intolerable cough (caused by elevated bradykinin).

Diuretics

Usually a thiazide-type diuretic is used (e.g. bendrofluazide). These drugs inhibit sodium reabsorption in the distal renal tubule, which causes increased salt and water excretion, decreasing blood volume and decreasing blood pressure. Side effects in high doses are:

- Hypokalaemia (low K$^+$) leading to arrhythmia and muscle fatigue.
- Hyperuricaemia (high uric acid) causing gout.
- Hyperglycaemia (raised blood glucose).
- Increased low-density lipoprotein (LDL) and very low-density lipoprotein (VLDL) leading to atherosclerosis.

Beta-blockers

Beta-blockers are antagonists of β-adrenoceptors. They block sympathetic activity in the heart (β$_1$), peripheral vasculature (β$_2$), and bronchi (β$_2$).

In the heart, this effect decreases heart rate and myocardial contractility. This results in a fall in cardiac output. Renin release from the juxtaglomerular cells is reduced and there is a central action, reducing sympathetic drive. These effects combine to lower blood pressure, but only in hypertensive patients.

The effect of β-blockers on the peripheral vasculature leads to a loss of β-mediated vasodilatation causing an unopposed α-vasoconstriction. This may initially cause an increase in vascular resistance, elevating blood pressure, but, in long-term use, the vascular resistance returns to pretreatment levels. However, peripheral blood flow may still be reduced, leading patients to complain of cold extremities.

Some β-blockers can preferentially act on β$_1$-adrenoceptors, being more cardioselective; however, even these drugs have some blocking effect on the β$_2$-adrenoceptor, and they should be given to asthmatic patients with extreme caution.

Types of β-blockers include:
- Propranolol (act on β$_1$, β$_2$).
- Metoprolol, atenolol, bisoprolol (selective β$_1$-blockers).

The main side effects of β-blockers are:
- Bronchoconstriction, leading to worsening asthma or chronic obstructive airways disease.
- Bradycardia.
- Hypoglycaemia.
- Fatigue and lethargy.
- Impotence.
- Sleep disturbance, nightmares, and vivid dreams (particularly propranolol).
- Rebound hypertension if stopped suddenly.

Many drugs of the same type have similar suffixes to their names. For example, most β-blockers end in '-ol' (e.g. propranolol, atenolol, metoprolol). This is useful when identifying the type of an unfamilar drug.

Alpha-blockers

Alpha-blockers (e.g. prazosin and doxazosin) are antagonists of α-adrenoceptors. There is postsynaptic block of α_1-adrenoceptors, which prevents sympathetic tonic drive and leads to vasodilatation. Therefore, there is a decrease in total peripheral resistance and thus a decrease in blood pressure. Doxazosin is often used for labile (catecholamine-mediated) hypertension.

Side effects of α-blockers are:

- Postural hypotension caused by loss of sympathetic vasoconstriction.
- First-dose phenomenon of rapid hypotension when initially administered.

Other sympatholytics

Adrenergic neuron blockers (e.g. guanethidine) prevent the release of noradrenaline from postganglionic neurons. They are rarely used now because they affect supine blood pressure control, and they may cause postural hypotension. They may be useful with other therapy in resistant hypertension.

Centrally acting α_2-agonists (e.g. methyldopa) decrease central sympathetic drive by displacing noradrenaline with a false transmitter (e.g. methylnoradrenaline from methyldopa). Release of the false transmitter is more active on α_2 pre-synaptic negative feedback receptors than α_1, reducing transmitter release and ultimately blood pressure. They are used to treat hypertension in pregnancy because more modern drugs have never been tested in pregnancy.

Calcium antagonists

Calcium antagonists (e.g. verapamil, nifedipine, amlodipine, diltiazem) block voltage-gated calcium channels in myocardium and vascular smooth muscle. This causes a decrease in myocardial contractility and electrical conductance and decreased vascular tone.

Calcium antagonists interfere with the action of various vasoconstrictor agonists (e.g. noradrenaline, angiotensin II, thrombin). All may precipitate heart failure (but this risk is reduced with nifedipine and nifedipine-like drugs, e.g. amlodipine).

Verapamil decreases cardiac output and heart rate (anti-arrhythmic activity), but it should not be used with β-blockers as it causes hypotension and asystole. The main side effect of verapamil is constipation.

Nifedipine and amlodipine relax vascular smooth muscle, dilating arteries. The main side effects are headache and ankle oedema.

Diltiazem also decreases vascular tone. This is often effective in angina. Its main side effect is bradycardia.

Potassium channel agonists

Potassium channel agonists (e.g. minoxidil and diazoxide) open ATP-dependent K^+ channels. Opening of K^+ channels hyperpolarizes vascular smooth muscle cells thereby making depolarization harder to achieve. This reduces the stimulation by vasoconstricting agonists on the muscle cells.

Potassium channel agonists are used only in severe hypertension when other methods have failed (diazoxide is used in hypertensive emergencies). They are usually used with a β-blocker and thiazide diuretic to counteract side effects.

Side effects of potassium channel agonists are:

- Increased hair growth (with minoxidil).
- Salt and water retention, leading to oedema (use thiazide).
- Reflex sympathetic activation causing tachycardia (use β-blocker).

Sodium nitroprusside

Sodium nitroprusside is an inorganic nitrate with a powerful vasodilator effect. It spontaneously breaks down into nitric oxide (NO), causing vascular smooth muscle relaxation. Sodium nitroprusside should only be used intravenously to control severe hypertensive crises (acute emergency situations). The side effects are excessive hypotension and cyanide toxicity (cyanide is a metabolite, causing tachycardia, metabolic acidosis, and arrhythmia—give sodium nitrite and sodium thiocyanate).

Combinations

ACE inhibitors are being used increasingly as a first-line treatment for hypertension as they carry a reduced risk of side effects. They can be combined with thiazide treatment, but caution should be used with existing diuretic treatment due to the risk of a collapse in blood pressure in volume depleted patients. Beta-blockers have traditionally been used with a thiazide if a thiazide has not been effective alone.

After these options have failed or are contraindicated, calcium antagonists should be tried. Diuretics may be used in addition, but verapamil should not be combined with β-blockers.

In severe hypertension where the above therapies have been tried or are contraindicated, then the vasodilators, α-blockers, and centrally acting drugs may be used. They may be used in conjunction with an ACE inhibitor, or a thiazide and a β-blocker, although doxazosin is being used more frequently in preference to diuretics and β-blockers because of its vasodilator effect and minimal side effects.

The adverse effects of drugs can usually be divided into types A and B.
- Type A effects are predictable.
- Type B effects are idiosyncratic.

For example, hypotension as a side effect of β-blockers is predictable, as their action is to decrease blood pressure—this is a type A effect. However, skin rashes occur as a hypersensitivity reaction—this would be a type B effect.

Lipids and the cardiovascular system

Lipid transport and metabolism
The insolubility of lipids in plasma means a special transport mechanism is required. This is provided by lipid–protein complexes known as lipoproteins, while the individual proteins are known as apolipoproteins. The apolipoproteins also act as receptors for cell surface proteins, which determine the destination of different lipoproteins. Low-density lipoprotein (LDL) is the main lipoprotein involved in the transport of cholesterol. Fig. 5.5 shows the main transport pathways for lipids from the diet (exogenous) and for lipids from the body's stores (endogenous).

It is thought that lipoprotein A is a prothrombotic lipoprotein that is particularly involved in coronary disease, while high levels of high-density lipoprotein (HDL) are protective. The classification of lipoproteins is outlined in Fig. 5.6.

Hyperlipidaemia
Hyperlipidaemia (Fig. 5.7) can be classified as hypertriglyceridaemia (raised triglycerides—also called triacylglycerides), hypercholesterolaemia (raised cholesterol), or hyperlipoproteinaemia (raised lipoproteins).

Effects of hyperlipidaemia
Atherosclerosis
There is a strong correlation between cholesterol levels and death rates from ischaemic vascular disease. There is an even stronger correlation between fibrinogen levels and ischaemic vascular disease. It must, therefore, be remembered that atherosclerosis is a multifactorial disease.

It is thought that LDL damages the arterial wall by producing oxygen radicals, or exacerbates wall injury from other causes. This may be opposed by the administration of antioxidants (e.g. vitamin E). Atheromatous plaques may develop in this damaged arterial wall.

Atherosclerosis occurs at a young age in some familial hyperlipidaemias, but not others.

HDL protects against atherosclerosis.

Acute pancreatitis
Acute pancreatitis can result from hypertriglyceridaemia.

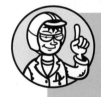

Hyperlipidaemias must be remembered as controllable causes of coronary heart disease, especially in the young.

Xanthomas
These are painful deposits of lipids in the skin and in tendons. They are usually diagnostic of hyperlipidaemia.

Treatment of hyperlipidaemia
Hyperlipidaemia can be treated by diet or drugs.

Dietary treatment involves reduction of calorific intake, saturated fats, cholesterol, and alcohol; supplements of omega-3 fats (present in fish oils) are given, increasing HDL levels, which is beneficial.

Indications for drug therapy are:
- High LDL levels, which must be treated if arterial disease is present.
- High triglycerides, which need to be treated only if symptomatic (e.g. causing xanthomas or pancreatitis).
- Low HDL levels.

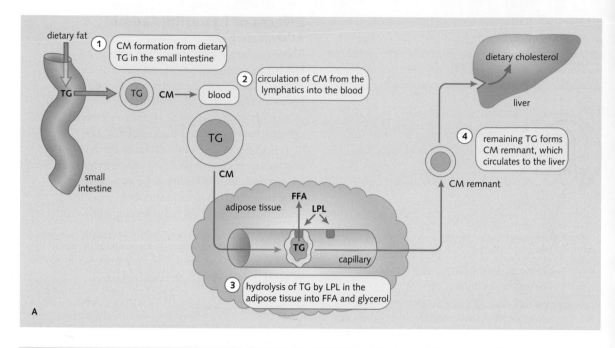

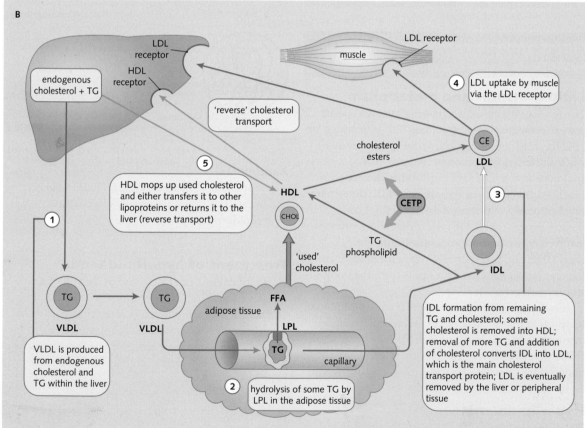

Fig. 5.5 (A) Exogenous and (B) endogenous lipid transport pathways. (CE, cholesterol esters; CETP, cholesterol ester transfer protein; CM, chylomicron; FFA, free fatty acid; HDL, high-density lipoprotein; IDL, intermediate-density lipoprotein; LDL, low-density lipoprotein; LPL, lipoprotein lipase; TG, triacylglycerol; VLDL, very low-density lipoprotein.)

Classification of lipoproteins		
Particle	Source	Predominantly transports
Chylomicron (CM)	Gut	Triacylglycerol
Very low-density lipoprotein (VLDL)	Liver	Triacylglycerol
Intermediate-density lipoprotein (IDL)	Catabolism	Cholesterol
Low-density lipoprotein (LDL)	Catabolism	Cholesterol
High-density lipoprotein (HDL)	Catabolism	Cholesterol
Lipoprotein A	Liver, gut	—

Fig. 5.6 Classification of lipoproteins.

Drugs used to lower triglyceride levels
Nicotinic acid
Nicotinic acid inhibits VLDL synthesis by the liver, leading to a decrease in intermediate density lipoprotein (IDL) and LDL. It also increases lipoprotein lipase (LPL) activity.

Nicotinic acid can be used for most types of hyperlipidaemia, usually in conjunction with a resin (see below). Its main side effects are rashes, nausea, abnormal liver function, and a prostaglandin-mediated cutaneous reaction. Its use has declined in favour of a statin (e.g. simvastatin).

Fibrates
Gemfibrozil reduces lipolysis of triglycerides in adipose tissue, leading to decreased hepatic production of VLDL. Bezafibrate increases LPL activity, which leads to decreased VLDL and decreased triglycerides, but it may increase LDL.

Classification of hyperlipidaemias					
Condition	Elevated lipoprotein	Elevated lipid	Biochemical defect	Drug therapy	Prevalence
Single gene defect					
Familial lipoprotein lipase (LPL) deficiency (type I)	CMs	Triacylglyceride	Low or absent LPL activity	Diet alone	Rare
Familial hypercholesterolaemia (type IIa)	LDL	Cholesterol	Deficiency of LDL receptors (none in homozygotes)	Statin, resin	Common
Familial combined hyperlipidaemia (type IIb)	VLDL, LDL	Triacylglyceride, cholesterol	Overproduction of apo-B	Fibrate	Common
Familial hyperlipoproteinaemia (type III)	CM remnants, IDL	Triacylglyceride, cholesterol	Abnormal apo-E	Fibrate	Rare
Familial hypertriglyceridaemia (type IV)	VLDL	Triacylglyceride	Overproduction of VLDL by the liver	Fibrate	Common
Familial hypertriglyceridaemia (type V)	VLDL, CMs	Triacylglyceride, cholesterol	Overproduction of VLDL by the liver	Fibrate	Rare
Multifactorial					
Hypertriglyceridaemia	VLDL	Triacylglyceride	Unknown	Fibrate	Common
Hypercholesterolaemia	LDL	Cholesterol	Unknown	Statin, resin	Common

Fig. 5.7 Classification of hyperlipidaemias. Familial, heritable abnormalities of lipid metabolism are classified according to Fredrickson type (types I–V) on the underlying genetic mutations. Hyperlipidaemia may also be multifactorial or idiopathic, without a currently identified or discrete genetic basis. These are clinically the most common in older patients. (CM, chylomicron; IDL, intermediate-density lipoprotein; LDL, low-density lipoprotein; VLDL, very low-density lipoprotein.)

Fibrates are used mainly in familial type III hyperlipidaemia. Gemfibrozil is the better drug as it does not increase LDL. The main side effects include nausea, abdominal discomfort and flu-like symptoms.

Drugs used to lower cholesterol
Bile acid binding resins (e.g. colestipol and cholestyramine)
Colestipol and cholestyramine inhibit reabsorption of cholesterol in the gut. They bind to bile salts in the gut and stop their reabsorption. This leads to increased excretion and decreased absorption of cholesterol. To compensate, the liver increases cholesterol conversion into bile salts and also increases LDL receptors. This removes LDL–cholesterol from circulation. They can aggravate hypertriglyceridaemia.

Statins (e.g. simvastatin and pravastatin)
Simvastatin and pravastatin are β-hydroxy-β-methylglutaryl coenzyme A (HMG CoA) reductase inhibitors. The liver compensates for the decreased cholesterol synthesis by increasing LDL receptors, which decreases plasma levels of LDL–cholesterol. They are used to treat most hypercholesterolaemias, and they are very effective if used in conjunction with a resin (up to 50% reduction in cholesterol levels). They are currently the only lipid-lowering treatment for which there is good evidence for reduced mortality.

The main side effects include reversible myositis and disturbed liver function tests.

Probucol
Probucol causes a 10% reduction in LDL–cholesterol, but it also lowers HDL and remains in the body for months. It has some antioxidant activity, which may reduce atherosclerosis formation.

Arteriosclerosis and atherosclerosis

Definitions and concepts
Arteriosclerosis is a term used to describe hardening and thickening of arteries. This reduces their elastic properties. Atherosclerosis is one of the processes that produces arteriosclerosis. It involves the formation of atheroma, which is an accumulation of lipid plaques within the walls of a vessel. Arteriosclerosis of small arteries and arterioles is termed arteriolosclerosis, and it is mainly caused by hypertension.

There are three main types of arteriosclerosis:
- Atherosclerosis.
- Arteriolosclerosis.
- Monckeberg's calcific medial sclerosis.

Consequences of arteriosclerosis
Arteriosclerosis results in a reduced arterial lumen with a consequent loss in perfusion. Furthermore, due to the loss of elasticity, rupture is more likely. There is also a predisposition to thrombus formation.

Atherosclerosis
It has been said that every adult in the Western world has some degree of atheroma in their arteries. Atherosclerosis and its complications are the main cause of mortality (over 50%) in the Western world. The incidence of atherosclerosis is rising in the UK.

Risk factors
Risk factors for atherosclerosis include constitutional factors such as:
- Age. Increased age increases the number and severity of lesions.
- Male sex. Men are affected to a much greater extent than women, until the menopause when the incidence in women increases, but men continue to be predominantly affected. This is thought to be because of the protective effect of oestrogens.
- Genetic predisposition.

Strong risk factors for atherosclerosis are:
- Smoking.
- Hypertension.
- Diabetes mellitus (see below).
- Hyperlipidaemia. It is directly related to levels of cholesterol and LDL. HDL levels are protective.
- Hyperfibrinogenaemia.
- Hyperhomocysteinaemia.

Other factors involved in the development of atherosclerosis are:
- Exercise—decreases the incidence of coronary heart disease; however, whether it prevents atheroma formation is unclear.
- Obesity—increases mortality, but this may only be a reflection of diet and lipid profile.
- Diet—decreased saturated fat intake has a beneficial effect, as may antioxidants (e.g. vitamin E in red wine).

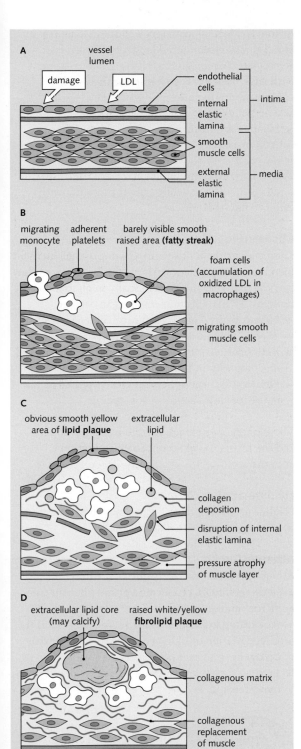

Fig. 5.8 Stages in the formation of an atheromatous plaque. (A) Damage to the endothelium. Chronic or repeated endothelial cell (EC) injury occurs, leading to metabolic dysfunction and structural changes. EC have a major role in actively preventing thrombus formation. Damage activates EC, upregulating inflammatory adhesion molecules (e.g. ICAM–1) and promoting monocyte and platelet adhesion. Injury also increases permeability to lipids and low-density lipoprotein (LDL) allowing movement into the intima. (B) Formation of a fatty streak. Monocytes adhere to the endothelium, migrate into the intima and become macrophages. There, they take up the LDL and become foam cells as they cannot degrade lipids. Local oxidation of LDL aids uptake by, and is chemotactic for, macrophages. Platelets adhere to activated endothelial cells or areas of denuded matrix. Activated platelets, activated EC and macrophages release platelet-derived growth factor (PDGF) and induce smooth muscle migration into the intima. (C) Development of lipid plaque. Smooth muscle proliferation and an increase in extracellular matrix occur in the intima. Smooth muscle cells also take up LDL and form foam cells. Greater macrophage infiltration takes place. Lipid may also be released free into the intima. Macrophages contribute many other factors (e.g. superoxide, proteases) that increase the damage. (D) Complicated plaques. As the lesion develops, pressure causes the media to atrophy and the muscle to be replaced by collagen. A fibrous cap of collagen forms on top. There is increased free lipid in the intima. The endothelium becomes fragile and ulcerates, leading to further platelet aggregation and thrombus formation.

Pathogenesis

Atherosclerosis generally affects medium to large arteries. It is characterized by lipid deposition in the intima, with smooth muscle and matrix proliferation combining to produce a fibrous plaque that protrudes into the lumen (Fig. 5.8). The lesions tend to be focal, patchy, and not involve the whole circumference of the vessel.

Certain stages (Fig. 5.8) are postulated to occur in atheroma formation according to the 'response to injury' hypothesis.

Other theories of pathogenesis include:
- Neoplasia. An abnormal proliferation of smooth muscle occurs, caused by some as yet unidentified factor that produces uncontrolled growth.
- Prostaglandins. The balance between prostacyclin and thromboxane has an influence on thrombus formation and, because fibrin and platelets are important components of atheromatous lesions, this must have a strong influence on pathogenesis.
- Thrombosis is the primary event that builds up in layers and organizes to form atheromatous plaques.

- Stress and personality—certain highly stressed and type A personalities may have an increased tendency to atherosclerosis and coronary heart disease.

Atherosclerosis is primarily an inflammatory process, and it is asymptomatic until it produces:

- Narrowing of the lumen—sufficient narrowing of the vessel produces symptoms of ischaemia (e.g. intermittent claudication, angina or gangrene).
- Sudden occlusion—caused by plaque rupture followed by thrombosis (e.g in myocardial infarction).
- Emboli—these may impact in other vessels.
- Aneurysms—resulting from wall weakening.

There is a high mortality associated with the formation of atheromatous plaques. A knowledge of how an atheroma is thought to occur is, therefore, expected in exams.

Treatment

The majority of research has looked at ways of reducing ischaemic heart disease by treating risk factors; it is not known what effect this has on the progress of atherosclerosis, but indirectly the following treatments have been used:

- Dietary control (reduced fat and sugar intake; increased amounts of fresh fruit and vegetables).
- Regular exercise and change in life-style (decrease stress).
- Stopping smoking.
- Cholesterol-lowering drugs (e.g. statins).

Monckeberg's medial calcific sclerosis

Monckeberg's medial calcific sclerosis is an idiopathic, degenerative disease of the elderly (aged over 50 years) characterized by focal calcifications in the media of small- and medium-sized arteries.

The femoral, tibial, radial, and ulnar arteries are predominantly involved. There is little or no inflammation, and usually the calcifications do not cause either obstructions or symptoms. There is an increase in pulse pressure (systolic hypertension) caused by loss of elasticity in the arteries.

Effects of diabetes mellitus on vessels

Diabetes mellitus causes a range of serious vascular complications, the severity of which is directly related to blood glucose levels. Intensive control of blood glucose (monitored long term by levels of glycosylated haemoglobin, HbA_{1c}), and treatment with ACE inhibitors can minimize these risks. Complications include:

- Microangiopathy.
- Hyaline arteriosclerosis.
- Atherosclerosis.

Type I diabetes is predominantly associated with small vessel disease, while type II predominantly causes large vessel disease.

Microangiopathy

Microangiopathy is diffuse thickening of the basement membranes of capillaries; paradoxically, however, they become more permeable, especially to plasma proteins. This results in specific organ damage:

- Nephropathy—glomerular involvement leads to microalbuminuria and can progress to renal failure.
- Retinopathy—degenerative changes include maculopathy and cataracts.
- Neuropathy—peripheral nerves, especially those in the lower leg are most susceptible.

These phenomena are related to hyperglycaemia and the formation of advanced glycosylation endproducts.

Hyaline arteriosclerosis

Hyaline arteriosclerosis is more prevalent and more severe in patients with diabetes mellitus.

Atherosclerosis

Atherosclerosis begins early during the onset of diabetes mellitus. Complicated plaques become more numerous and severe. Contributing factors include:

- Associated hyperlipidaemia and decreased HDL.
- Glycosylation of LDL and its cross-linking with collagen.
- Increased platelet adhesion caused by obesity and hypertension.

There is a greater incidence of ischaemic heart disease among people with diabetes mellitus than for the rest of the population. Do not forget that diabetes mellitus is a very major risk factor.

Aneurysms

Definitions and concepts

An aneurysm is an abnormal, localized, permanent dilatation of an artery or part of the heart (Fig. 5.9). It is caused by weakening of the wall:

- A true aneurysm is surrounded by all three layers of the arterial wall.
- A false aneurysm occurs when there is an actual hole in all or part of the arterial wall, which causes blood to move extravascularly, producing a haematoma. A dissecting aneurysm occurs when the blood is contained between the internal layers of the arterial wall and progresses by splitting the muscular layers (Fig. 5.10).

Aneurysms are caused by:

- Atherosclerosis. Plaque formation causes medial destruction and wall thinning. This commonly occurs in the abdominal aorta.
- Cystic medial degeneration—mucinous degeneration of the media with fragmentation of the elastic tissue. This is often seen in dissecting aortic aneurysms.
- Syphilis.
- Trauma.
- Vasculitides (especially polyarteritis nodosa).

- Congenital defects (e.g. berry aneurysms).
- Infections (mycotic aneurysms).

Aneurysms are often described by their shape. They are either fusiform (spindle shaped, being tapered at either end) or saccular (sac-like).

Mycotic aneurysms are aneurysms caused by infection. Bacteria within septic emboli that lodge in arteries may cause destruction of the arterial wall.

Turbulence of blood within an aneurysm frequently leads to the formation of a thrombus, increasing the risk of rupture.

Abdominal aortic aneurysm

The prevalence of abdominal aortic aneurysms is 3% in men aged over 50 years.

The aneurysm is usually found proximal to the iliac bifurcation of the abdominal aorta. The patient may be asymptomatic or have abdominal/back pain.

Leaking and rupture with resultant haemorrhage is the most serious complication. Fistulae into the gut or vena cava may rarely occur.

Hypertension increases the risk of rupture, and 30% of abdominal aortic aneurysms will rupture. Risk of rupture increases with larger aneurysms.

Surgery aims to prevent rupture. Elective surgery has an operative mortality of 5%. Operative mortality rises to 50% if the aneurysm ruptures. Treatment aims to replace the aneurysm with a Dacron graft. Postoperative complications include myocardial infarction and renal failure.

Syphilitic (luetic) aneurysm

Syphilitic (luetic) aneurysms can occur in the thoracic aorta of patients with tertiary syphilis.

There is inflammation of the adventitia, especially the vasa vasorum (endarteritis). This causes ischaemia and loss of muscle and elastic tissue, which leads to weakening of the arterial wall.

Microscopically the vasa vasorum have thickened walls, and they are surrounded by inflammatory cells. The aneurysm may extend backwards along the aorta to the aortic valve leading to valve regurgitation.

Sequelae include syphilitic heart disease, compression of adjacent structures, and rupture.

Aortic dissection

In this condition, blood in the aorta is dissected into two flows: one in the normal lumen and another in one of the layers of the media (Fig. 5.10). An intimal

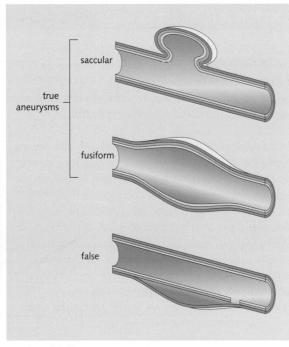

Fig. 5.9 Types of aneurysm: saccular, fusiform, and false.

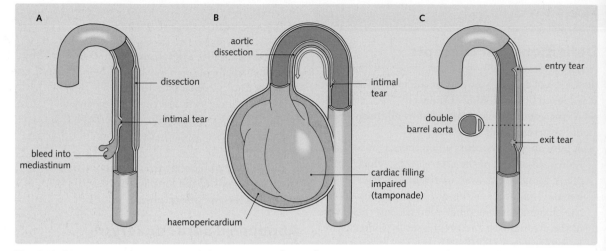

Fig. 5.10 Dissecting aortic aneurysm. (A) Rupture into the mediastinum. (B) Rupture into the pericardium. (C) Rupture into the aorta.

tear usually occurs in the ascending aorta within 10 cm of the aortic valve, creating an entry point for blood to move into one of the fascial layers of the wall.

Aortic dissection is seen predominantly in men aged 40–60 years with systemic hypertension, and it commonly occurs in Marfan syndrome, where cystic medial degeneration occurs. It may also occur as a result of trauma, especially iatrogenic (e.g. during arterial cannulation).

Clinical features include sudden onset of severe chest pain radiating to the back and downwards.

Sequelae of dissection include:
- Rupture into the thorax or abdomen.
- Occlusion of aortic branches, especially coronary, cerebral, and renal arteries.
- Extension along the aorta to include other arteries or disruption of the aortic valve.
- Cardiac tamponade caused by extension and rupture into the pericardium.

Other causes of aneurysms
Congenital causes
Berry aneurysms in the circle of Willis can be caused by focal weakness in the arterial wall of the cerebral vessels. These occasionally rupture, leading to subarachnoid haemorrhage.

Vasculitides
Two forms of vasculitis may cause aneurysm (see p. 103):
- Polyarteritis nodosa. Aneurysms may form in any organ with vessels affected by the disease.

- Kawasaki syndrome. Dilatation of the coronary arteries associated with arteritis is a complication of the disease.

Myocardial ischaemia
Myocardial ischaemia may lead to dilatation and aneurysm of the ventricle. This may later rupture. A similar aneurysm may also occur in Chagas' disease (trypanosomiasis).

Ischaemic heart disease

Ischaemic heart disease occurs when the blood supply to the myocardium is insufficient for its needs. This can be due to:
- An impaired blood supply to the myocardium.
- An increased demand by the myocardium.

Ischaemia can also occur because of reduced oxygen transport (e.g in shock, severe anaemia, lung disease, and congenital heart disease) and may contribute significantly to damage if it occurs with the above.

Ischaemic heart disease (also called coronary heart disease) is the leading cause of death in the Western world (30% of male and 23% of female deaths). It is mainly caused by atherosclerosis of the coronary arteries, and more commonly affects the left ventricle because of its larger size and demand. The main clinical syndromes are either chronic or acute.

Predisposing factors include:
- Hypercholesterolaemia.
- Smoking.

- Hypertension.
- Age.
- Male sex.
- Diabetes mellitus and insulin resistance.
- Family history of previous ischaemic heart disease.
- Prothrombotic factors (high fibrinogen, raised factor VII).
- Elevated homocysteine levels.
- Obesity.
- Excessive alcohol intake.
- Geography (high risk in Scotland, low risk in Sweden).
- Type A personality.
- Low socio-economic class.

The aetiology of ischaemic heart disease is usually a result of complications of atherosclerotic plaques in the coronary arteries, which can be:
- Progressive atherosclerosis leading to stenosis.
- Thrombus formation on a plaque caused by superficial ulceration.
- Plaque fissuring, leading to thrombus formation in the lumen or haemorrhage into the plaque.

Vasospasm may precipitate these changes or reduce coronary blood flow on its own (e.g. in Prinzmetal's angina). Ischaemia can also result from:
- Narrowing of the coronary ostia in syphilis or atherosclerosis.
- Emboli as a result of infective endocarditis.
- Coronary artery disease (e.g. polyarteritis nodosa).
- Shock caused by haemorrhage.
- Severe aortic valvular disease.
- Severe anaemia.

Chronic ischaemic heart disease

Chronic ischaemic heart disease occurs in elderly persons with severe atherosclerosis of many coronary vessels. Patients may progressively develop congestive cardiac failure. Atrophy of the myocytes and diffuse fibrosis can be seen microscopically. Death may be caused by:
- Cardiac failure.
- Acute myocardial infarction.
- Arrhythmia.

Acute ischaemic heart disease

Unstable angina (or crescendo angina) is a sudden onset of angina, caused by the fissuring of atherosclerotic plaques. Myocardial infarction occurs when a region of the myocardium fails to be perfused with blood and becomes necrotic.

Sudden cardiac death is usually caused by ventricular fibrillation, but it can be caused by an acute myocardial infarction.

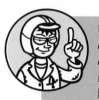 Unstable angina should be considered a medical emergency since it has a high mortality and it may rapidly lead to myocardial infarction. Rapid access to treatment will prevent this.

Angina pectoris

Angina pectoris is episodic pain that is usually induced by exercise, and it occurs in the centre of the chest, often radiating to the neck and left arm. It is commonly classified as:
- Angina of effort (classic angina)—occurs after exertion, excitation or emotion and is caused by an insufficient oxygen supply to meet an increased demand. Classically, the pain subsides with rest. It may be stable (gradual stenosis by a progressive plaque build-up) or unstable (sudden plaque fissuring producing thrombosis).
- Vasospastic (Prinzmetal's) angina—caused by transient spasm of the coronary artery obstructing blood flow. The spasm is probably mediated by α-receptors.

Angina occurs because myocardial oxygen requirement is greater than its supply. This leads to a build-up in local metabolites causing pain.

Treatment of angina

Treatment strategies for angina involve increasing oxygen supply to the ischaemic zone and decreasing oxygen demand by the myocardium. Increasing oxygen supply to the ischaemic zone can be achieved by dilating the coronary arteries or decreasing heart rate:
- Coronary arteries only supply blood during diastole. With a slower heart rate diastole is prolonged giving more time for perfusion of the myocardium.
- Dilating coronary arteries (e.g. Ca^{2+} antagonists) is useful in vasospastic angina. It has only a small effect on angina of effort as the coronary arteries are already fully dilated.

Decreasing the oxygen demand of the myocardium can be achieved by two methods:
- Directly decreasing force and heart rate (β-blockers, Ca^{2+} antagonists).
- Decreasing blood pressure and heart size and thus wall force by using vasodilators and venodilators (nitrates, nicorandil, Ca^{2+} antagonists; reduce load).

Active control of risk factors is also a key component of long-term management, and this should not be neglected (e.g. smoking cessation, regular exercise, and dietary control).

Organic nitrates

Organic nitrates, for example, glyceryl trinitrate (GTN), act by relaxing vascular smooth muscle by producing NO in smooth muscle, which increases cyclic guanosine monophosphate (cGMP) and brings about dilatation. The greatest effect is on venous capacitance vessels, increasing venous pooling and, therefore, reducing heart size, wall force, and myocardial oxygen demand.

Organic nitrates are used in both angina of effort and vasospastic angina:
- Angina of effort. By Starling's law, decreased venous return results in decreased cardiac output and, therefore, oxygen demand.
- Vasospastic angina. They have a direct dilatory effect on the coronary arteries, reducing spasm.

GTN is subject to first-pass metabolism, and it is, therefore, taken sublingually. The effect lasts for approximately 30 min. It is used to stop or prevent an angina attack. Longer acting nitrates include isosorbide mononitrate and isosorbide dinitrate. Side effects are:
- Postural or systemic hypotension.
- Reflex tachycardia.
- Headache and facial flushing.
- Tolerance (may develop over 2–3 days continuous use).

Calcium channel blockers (e.g. nifedipine, verapamil, diltiazem)

These drugs block Ca^{2+} channels, decreasing contraction of smooth and cardiac muscle. Nifedipine acts more on smooth muscle than cardiac muscle. They mainly cause vasodilatation, and they are used in both angina of effort and vasospastic angina:
- Angina of effort. Calcium channel blockers decrease total peripheral resistance, lessening the demand on the heart.

- Vasospastic angina. These drugs cause relaxation of spasm.

Side effects of calcium channel blockers are:
- Headache and facial flushing.
- Constipation.
- Reflex tachycardia.
- Oedema.

Verapamil should not be combined with β-blockers, while nifedipine may be beneficially combined with β-blockers to minimize reflex tachycardia.

Potassium channel openers

Potassium channel openers (e.g. nicorandil) act by opening ATP-dependent K^+ channels in vascular smooth muscle, making depolarization more difficult to achieve and leading to vasodilatation and venodilation. This reduces heart size, wall force, and myocardial oxygen demand.

Potassium channel openers are an alternative to nitrates when tolerance occurs and if β-blockers and Ca^{2+} antagonists are contraindicated. Nicorandil has some nitrate effects. Side effects are:
- Headache and facial flushing.
- Postural hypotension.
- Weakness.

Beta-blockers

These drugs block sympathetic stimulation of the heart, leading to:
- Decreased force and, therefore, decreased oxygen demand.
- Decreased rate and, therefore, decreased oxygen demand and also increased time for oxygen supply.

They are used in angina of effort, but not in vasospastic angina as they have no dilatory effect. They should not be used to treat patients with asthma, peripheral arterial disease, or bradyarrhythmias.

 The mechanism and treatment of angina are frequently asked about in examination questions.

Myocardial infarction

Myocardial infarction is classified as:
- Subendocardial myocardial infarction—affecting the innermost region of the myocardium.

- Regional myocardial infarction—affecting the full thickness of one segment of the myocardium.

Myocardial infarction occurs when an area of muscle of the heart dies (i.e. undergoes necrosis). It is caused by a reduction or blockage in the coronary blood supply, and it is usually precipitated by thrombosis or haemorrhage in an atherosclerotic area of a coronary artery. There are many complications including arrhythmias, heart failure, and even sudden death.

Subendocardial myocardial infarction

This is an infarction of the subendocardial layer of the myocardium. Diffuse atherosclerosis is present in all three main arteries. The infarction is caused by either:

- Increased demand.
- Hypotension.
- Vasospasm.

It may not involve a superimposed thrombosis. Injury is less severe than that of transmural infarcts and can be diffuse or regional.

Transmural myocardial infarction

A transmural infarction affects the full thickness of the myocardium. It usually involves an occlusion of a major coronary artery, causing ischaemia to a specific region of the heart. Transmural myocardial infarction may be caused by:

- An acute plaque change (ulceration, fissuring, or haemorrhage) leading to thrombosis.
- Platelet aggregation.
- Vasospasm (rarely).

Complete occlusion of a vessel may not cause infarction as collaterals may have developed, aiding perfusion.

Nearly all infarcts affect the left ventricle; 15% involve both ventricles, and 3% involve just the right ventricle. The arteries commonly infarcted are:

- Left anterior descending artery (50%)—affecting the left ventricular anterior wall and interventricular septum.
- Right coronary artery (30%)—affecting the left ventricular inferior and posterior walls and right ventricle.
- Left circumflex artery (20%)—affecting the left ventricular lateral wall.

From the onset of ischaemia, it takes only 20–40 minutes until irreversible injury starts to occur. Reperfusion (the return of flow) caused by thrombolysis (spontaneous or drug-induced) can lessen the extent of damage. Reperfused myocytes may not function to the same level for a few days. A characteristic series of events occurs (Fig. 5.11).

Sudden death occurs in 25% of patients, usually as a result of an arrhythmia; 90% of survivors develop acute or chronic complications. Acute complications include:

- Arrhythmias.
- Heart failure.
- Cardiogenic shock.
- Ventricular rupture.
- Papillary muscle infarction, leading to mitral valve incompetence.
- Mural thrombosis, leading to pulmonary or peripheral thromboembolism.
- Pericarditis.

Chronic complications include:

- Ventricular aneurysm and thrombosis.
- Recurrent infarction.
- Arrhythmias.
- Chronic heart failure.

Mortality is 35% in the first year, and 10% every year thereafter.

Events occurring after myocardial infarction		
Time after myocardial infarction	Macroscopic events	Microscopic events
6–12 h	Normal	Oedema
12–18 h	Normal	Neutrophils appear
18–24 h	Pale or cyanotic	Myocyte necrosis
1–3 days	Hyperaemic border	Inflammation
3–7 days	Yellow, sharply defined lesion that softens	Dead cells disintegrate and are mopped up by macrophages
7–10 days	Haemorrhagic edge	Granulation tissue replaces dead tissue
12 days	Scar formation	Dense fibrous tissue

Fig. 5.11 Time line of events occurring after infarction.

Make sure you go to your pathology museum and place the pots of myocardial infarction exhibits in order of the time after infarction. This will help to reinforce the changes that occur after infarction.

Treatment

Fibrinolytic drugs

Thrombolytic (fibrinolytic) therapy is used to breakdown the thrombi that cause a myocardial infarction. If given within 3 hours, it probably allows reperfusion in about half of the affected arteries.

Thrombolytics include:

- Streptokinase—binds and activates plasminogen to form plasmin, causing fibrinolysis. Plasmin also lyses fibrinogen and prothrombin (anticoagulant effect). Streptokinase cannot be used repeatedly as it can cause anaphylactic reactions.
- Anistreplase (APSAC)—is metabolized to streptokinase.
- (Recombinant) tissue plasminogen activator— (r)tPA—used when streptokinase has been used recently in a previous myocardial infarction as it does not cause any allergic anaphylactic reactions. It is increasingly used in large anterior infarction in accordance with the results of the GUSTO trials (a series of global studies of cardiovascular disease treatments). It must be given with heparin.

Several trials have shown that all three fibrinolytic drugs are generally equally effective in the treatment of acute myocardial infarction, although the GUSTO trials have shown that tPA is more beneficial in high risk patients. Side effects are:

- Nausea and vomiting.
- Bleeding (may result in strokes).

Non-steroidal anti-inflammatory drugs (NSAIDs)

Aspirin is an NSAID that irreversibly inhibits the cyclooxygenase enzyme. It has been shown to be beneficial in an acute myocardial infarction (with streptokinase) and in preventing myocardial infarction and stroke.

Aspirin's beneficial effects in thromboembolic disease are thought to be caused by decreased synthesis of thromboxane A_2 (Tx-A_2) by platelets. Tx-A_2 is a strong inducer of platelet aggregation. Its action is antagonized by prostacyclin (PGI$_2$) from endothelial cells. PGI$_2$ synthesis is also blocked by aspirin, but the endothelial cell is able to produce more cyclooxygenase enzyme (this cannot occur in platelets as they have no nucleus). The overall action, therefore, is to favour non-aggregation of platelets. Side effects are:

- Bronchospasm.
- Gastrointestinal haemorrhage.

Sudden cardiac death

Sudden cardiac death is unexpected death from a cardiac cause within 1 hour of onset of symptoms. There is usually plaque disruption, but ultimately death is caused by a fatal arrhythmia (asystole or ventricular fibrillation) due to scarring of the conduction system, acute ischaemic injury, or electrolyte imbalance.

Heart failure

Definition

Heart failure (cardiac failure) is said to have occurred when the heart is no longer able to maintain the circulation to the tissues for normal metabolism.

Conditions

Conditions that lead to heart failure can be divided into:

- Those that damage cardiac muscle (e.g. ischaemic heart disease, cardiomyopathies).
- Those that demand extra work of the heart (e.g. systemic hypertension, valvular heart disease).

Symptoms and signs

Symptoms and signs of heart failure are:

- Muscle fatigue.
- Reduced exercise tolerance.
- Tachycardia.
- Dyspnoea, possibly caused by increased fluid in the lungs.
- Orthopnoea (shortness of breath while lying flat).
- Paroxysmal nocturnal dyspnoea (sudden shortness of breath while sleeping).
- Haemoptysis caused by increased venous pressure, leading to alveolar haemorrhage.
- Elevated jugular venous pressure (due to venous congestion).
- Hepatomegaly (due to venous congestion).
- Oedema (due to venous congestion).
- Proteinuria caused by prerenal renal failure.

Remember, 'heart failure' is NOT a diagnosis. You must ALWAYS identify the underlying pathology that is responsible.

Compensatory mechanisms

There is a decrease in contractility of the affected heart muscle in chronic heart failure. This shifts the Starling curve to the right and reduces the force of contraction for a given filling pressure (Fig. 5.12). The body attempts to compensate by increasing filling pressure (Fig. 5.13).

This is achieved by:

- Catecholamine release causing increased sympathetic nerve activity, increasing heart rate and force.
- Peripheral vasoconstriction/venoconstriction, which will increase filling pressure but also total peripheral resistance (this increases the demand on the heart).
- Renal retention of Na^+ and water to increase blood volume and filling pressure, also causing oedema.

These responses only confer a limited improvement. Increased cardiac filling initially increases cardiac

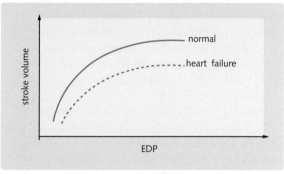

Fig. 5.12 The Starling curve in heart failure. Reduced contractility reduces stroke volume for a given filling pressure. (EDP, end-diastolic pressure.)

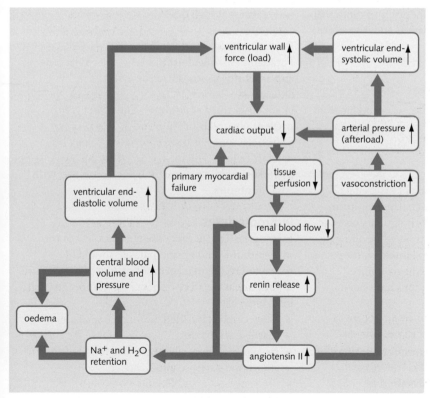

Fig. 5.13 The series of changes in heart failure is initiated by myocardial changes, which impair the efficiency of the heart. Causes include infarction, cardiomyopathy, and chronic hypertension. In the normal heart, an increased end-diastolic or systolic volume leads to greater cardiac output by Starling's law, but in a heart with impaired contractility there is little further reserve. Dilatation of the ventricles further impairs the efficiency of the heart by Laplace's law, requiring greater effort to maintain output.

Compensatory changes include sympathetic activation to increase contractility and to raise blood pressure, in order to maintain tissue perfusion, but chronic stimulation leads to an impaired adrenergic response. The renin–angiotensin system is also activated, leading to fluid retention and raised blood pressure.

Attempts to raise the systemic blood pressure place further load on an already weakened heart, creating a destructive cycle. Therapy is aimed at controlling these compensatory mechanisms to unload the heart and prevent excessive dilatation.

output through Starling's law, but prolonged excessive cardiac filling causes excessive dilatation. This leads to ineffective contraction and causes the heart to enlarge (hypertrophy) and eventually fail. According to Laplace's law, dilatation of the heart requires the myocytes to increase the tension in the wall to sustain the same pressure (see p. 51). This increases oxygen demand and predisposes the myocardium to ischaemia. Dilatation may also ultimately lead to valvular incompetence. A key aim for treatment is, therefore, to reduce the load on the failing heart, for example, by venodilation, although this carries a risk of precipitating cardiogenic shock.

Increased catecholamine release (i.e. increased sympathetic drive) results in increased adrenaline and noradrenaline secretion to increase the force and rate of contraction. As the condition worsens, there is an eventual downregulation of β-adrenoceptors reducing this effect.

Treatment of heart failure
Angiotensin-converting enzyme inhibitors
ACE inhibitors (e.g. enalapril, lisinopril, and captopril):
- Block production of angiotensin II and, therefore, aldosterone.
- Prevent the breakdown of bradykinin.
- Prolong life in heart failure.

ACE inhibitors produce vasodilatation/venodilatation, thereby decreasing load and oedema. (ACE inhibitors are also used in hypertension, see p. 76).

Beta-blockers
The sympatholytic effects of β-blockers (see p. 77) have been shown to be beneficial in the long-term management of heart failure. Their action slows the heart, thereby increasing filling time while allowing β-receptor sensitivity to recover. However, they should not be used to treat acute heart failure.

Side effects and contraindications have been described previously (see p.77).

Diuretics
Diuretics increase salt and water excretion, therefore decreasing circulatory volume. This decreases preload and oedema. They are classified as:
- Thiazides.
- Loop diuretics.
- Potassium-sparing diuretics.

Thiazides are used in mild cardiac failure and hypertension (see p. 77); loop diuretics are used in moderate and severe heart failure; potassium-sparing diuretics are sometimes used in conjunction with other diuretics to prevent hypokalaemia.

Diuretics are often used in combination with an ACE inhibitor.

Thiazides
Thiazides (e.g. chlorothiazide, bendrofluazide, metolazone) prevent Na^+ and Cl^- reabsorption in the distal tubule. Side effects are:
- Hypokalaemia.
- Hyperuricaemia.
- Hypercholesterolaemia.
- Hyperglycaemia.

Loop diuretics
Loop diuretics (e.g. frusemide and bumetanide) inhibit NaCl reabsorption in the loop of Henle. They cause more potent diuresis than other diuretics, and they can be used in patients with reduced renal function. Side effects are:
- Those of thiazides.
- Deafness at high doses.

Potassium-sparing diuretics
Potassium-sparing diuretics (e.g. spironolactone and amiloride) antagonize the effect of aldosterone (spironolactone) or may block Na^+ channels in the distal tubule. The effect is to prevent Na^+ reabsorption and K^+ excretion. Spironolactone has been shown to prolong life in heart failure. The main side effect is hyperkalaemia, a major risk when combined with ACE inhibitors.

Inotropic drugs
Inotropic drugs increase the contractility of the myocardium. Their principal role should be restricted to the management of acute heart failure, as they are associated with increased mortality with long-term use.

They can be classified as:
- Cardiac glycosides.
- $β_1$-sympathomimetics.
- Phosphodiesterase inhibitors.

Cardiac glycosides
Cardiac glycosides (e.g. digoxin and ouabain) inhibit the sodium pump, which leads to a rise in intracellular Ca^{2+}. This:
- Increases the force of contraction.
- Reduces the heart's oxygen consumption.

They also have a central effect to increase vagal activity, which slows the heart rate.

The side effects of cardiac glycosides are:

- Anorexia.
- Nausea and vomiting.
- Diarrhoea.
- Confusion.
- Arrhythmia in toxic doses.

Cardiac glycosides are contraindicated in hypokalaemia because of potentiation of their action, and they should be combined with thiazides and loop diuretics with caution.

β_1-sympathomimetics

The β_1-sympathomimetics dobutamine and dopamine increase the force of contraction. Dopamine also increases renal blood flow in low doses. Side effects are tachycardia and hypertension in overdose.

Phosphodiesterase inhibitors (milrinone)

Milrinone (caffeine) inhibits phosphodiesterase, which is the enzyme that breaks down cyclic adenosine monophosphate (cAMP) into 5'-AMP. Inhibition causes a rise in intracellular cAMP and, therefore, Ca^{2+}. This means there is an increase in contractility. Milirone is also a vasodilator. It is used in severe heart failure that is unresponsive to other therapy.

Arrhythmia

Definitions and classification

An arrhythmia is any deviation from the heart's normal sinus rhythm. Descriptions of arrhthymias are outlined below. Arrhythmias are usually classified clinically as supraventricular or ventricular.

- Supraventricular—originating in the atrium or atrioventricular node.
- Ventricular—originating in the ventricle.

Altered sinus rhythms

Sinus tachycardia and sinus bradycardia are produced by autonomic nervous activity. It usually takes several beats to produce a new steady state.

Tachycardia (>100 beats/min in adults) usually results from:

- Exercise.
- Emotion.
- Fever.

Sinus tachycardia will show normal P waves, with a stable P–R interval within normal limits.

Bradycardia (<60 beats/min) commonly occurs in:

- Athletes.
- Patients with raised intracranial pressure.

Sinus arrhythmia generally manifests in the young as a change in rhythm with respiration. The heart rate increases with inspiration and decreases with expiration.

Extrasystole (ectopic beats)

Extrasystole occurs when an abnormal beat is generated in an area of myocardium before the next sinus beat. The impulse that is generated goes on to contract the ventricle. Atrial extrasystole or ventricular extrasystole may occur, depending upon the area of origin. Usually, there is a gap before the next normal sinus beat; this is termed the compensatory phase.

Atrial (supraventricular) tachycardia and atrial flutter

Atrial tachycardia and atrial flutter are caused by an abnormal focus in the atrium or an abnormal conduction pathway causing re-entry that results in atrial contraction at a rapid rate. It may also be caused by ectopic or junctional beats that may arise from the myocardium surrounding the atrioventricular node, or the tissue forming the 'junctional area' which connects the atrioventricular node to the ventricular conduction system. Ectopic beats, or abnormal conduction (eg. Wolff–Parkinson–White, ischaemia) within this area may produce an atrioventricular re-entry tachycardia. P waves may be inverted on an ECG, but they may still cause atrial or ventricular contraction.

In atrial flutter the rate is usually around 300 beats/min but not all atrial impulses are conducted to the ventricle. Often, the ratio of atrial to ventricular beats is 2:1 or 3:1 (i.e. a variable atrioventricular heart block, see below).

Supraventricular tachycardia is characterized by a heart rate between 140 and 220 beats/min, with narrow QRS complexes.

Atrial fibrillation

There is no coordinated atrial activity in atrial fibrillation. A rippling effect of the muscle occurs, which does not contribute to ventricular filling. Ventricular activity is affected, producing a characteristic 'irregularly irregular' pulse. It is commonly caused by mitral valve disease, ischaemic heart disease, or thyrotoxicosis.

Wolff–Parkinson–White syndrome

In Wolff–Parkinson–White syndrome, there is an extra conduction pathway (the bundle of Kent) between the atria and ventricles. This results in rapid conduction, which can lead to tachycardia or atrial fibrillation.

Heart block (atrioventricular block)

This is an interruption of the normal conduction through the atrioventricular conduction tissue. It may be classified as first-, second-, or third-degree block.

First-degree heart block

In first-degree heart block, all atrial impulses reach the ventricle, but conduction through the atrioventricular tissue takes longer than normal (P–R interval on an electrocardiogram is >0.2 s).

Second-degree heart block

In second-degree heart block, some atrial impulses fail to reach the ventricles, but others do (not all P waves are followed by QRS complexes).

Third-degree (complete) heart block

In third-degree heart block, the atria and ventricles beat independently of each other. The ventricular rate is usually about 20–40 beats/min (P waves and QRS complexes have no fixed relationship).

Wenckebach heart block

In Wenckebach heart block, the degree of block increases over a few beats (P–R interval increases over three or four beats, followed by an isolated P wave).

Ventricular tachycardia

Ventricular tachycardia occurs when impulses originate from an ectopic focus within the ventricles. It is characterized by broad QRS complexes (i.e. duration > 120 ms) on an ECG at a rate of > 120 beats/min. It is often a precursor to ventricular fibrillation.

Ventricular fibrillation

Ventricular fibrillation is an irregular uncoordinated rippling contraction of the ventricle. There is no effective cardiac output, leading to rapid loss of consciousness. Death results unless effective treatment is initiated immediately.

Mechanism of arrhythmia

Arrhythmias are caused by a combination of abnormal impulse generation (either an abnormal sinus rhythm or an ectopic pacemaker), delayed depolarization after an action potential (which can result in a second contraction), and re-entry. A more detailed account of arrhythmia is given in Chapter 8.

Anti-arrhythmic drugs

The aims of drug treatment are:
- To decrease cell excitability.
- To increase the refractory period.
- To slow conduction or block conduction if already slow.

The Vaughan–Williams classification system is used for anti-arrhythmic drugs; it is based on their actions.

Class I: sodium channel blockers

These drugs can be subdivided into class IA (e.g. quinidine, procainamide, and disopyramide), class IB (e.g. lignocaine, mexiletine, and tocainide), and class IC (e.g. flecainide). They block sodium channels during the open (classes IA and IC) or refractory (class IB) state. They are all 'use-dependent' blockers, only affecting active channels.

Class IA: quinidine, procainamide, disopyramide

Class IA drugs prolong the action potential by:
- Increasing the threshold for spontaneous depolarization.
- Slowing the fast upstroke.
- Prolonging the refractory period.

These drugs are used for supraventricular and ventricular arrhythmias. Side effects are:
- Nausea and vomiting.
- Anticholinergic effects—dry mouth, blurred vision, and urinary retention.
- Hypotension (disopyramide).
- Precipitation of systemic lupus erythematosus (procainamide).

Quinidine and procainamide should be used with caution due to risks of more severe side effects.

Class IB: lignocaine (lidocaine), mexiletine, tocainide

Class IB drugs bind preferentially to refractory Na^+ channels, and so they act preferentially on ischaemic myocardium. They shorten the action potential by:
- Slowing the fast upstroke.
- Increasing the refractory period.

They are used for ventricular arrhythmias, especially after a myocardial infarction. Side effects are:

- Convulsions.
- Nausea and vomiting.

Class IC: flecainide

Class IC drugs have little effect on action potential, but they slow upstroke and conduction speed; there is little change in refractory period. They are used in supraventricular and ventricular arrhythmias. Side effects are:

- Further arrhythmias.
- Dizziness.

Class II: β-adrenergic blockers

Class II drugs (e.g. propranolol and atenolol) block the increase in pacemaker activity that is produced by sympathetic stimulation of β-adrenoceptors. They also slow conduction.

Beta-blockers may be used for ectopic beats, atrial fibrillation, and atrial tachycardia. They are indicated when circulating catecholamines are too high (e.g. after a myocardial infarction and thyrotoxicosis). Side effects are:

- Tiredness.
- Provoke asthma.

Some drugs (such as sotalol and bretylium) have both class II and III actions.

Class III: potassium channel blockers

Class III drugs (e.g. amiodarone) block K^+ channels, slowing repolarization leading to a prolonged action potential and refractory period.

Class III drugs are used in supraventricular and ventricular arrhythmias. Side effects of amiodarone are:

- Photosensitivity (turn blue in sun).
- Liver damage.
- Thyroid disorders.
- Neuropathy.
- Pulmonary alveolitis.

Amiodarone also has class IA and II effects.

Class IV: calcium channel blockers

Class IV drugs (e.g. verapamil) block Ca^{2+} channels, thereby decreasing spontaneous activity and conduction at sinoatrial and atrioventricular nodes.

Class IV drugs are used for supraventricular arrhythmias only. Side effects of verapamil are:

- Precipitation of cardiac failure.

- Atrioventricular block.
- Constipation.

Other drugs not in this classification

These include:

- Digitalis (digoxin)—used for supraventricular arrhythmias, especially atrial fibrillation. It has a central effect, stimulating the vagus, causing partial atrioventricular block. This slows the ventricular beat and causes stronger contractions. It also inhibits Na^+/K^+ ATPase.
- Adenosine—used to terminate supraventricular tachycardias.
- Calcium chloride—used for broad-complex tachycardia.
- Magnesium chloride—used for ventricular fibrillation and to treat digoxin excess.
- Atropine—used to treat bradycardia. It acts by blocking parasympathetic effects on the heart.
- Adrenaline—used in cardiac arrest.
- Isoprenaline—used in the treatment of heart block while awaiting pacing.

Sicilian Gambit classification

In 1991, a group of basic and clinical investigators devised a new classification for anti-arrhythmic drugs. Anti-arrhythmic drugs fit awkwardly into the Vaughan–Williams classification because of their mixed actions. This new classification provides the best information available on the current anti-arrhythmic drugs based on their individual actions. This classification has taken over from the Vaughan–Williams classification. A spreadsheet of the actions of current medication has been published (Fig. 5.14).

Disorders of the heart valves

Heart valve disease produces two types of disorder: stenosis and regurgitation. Stenosis is an obstruction to the normal flow of blood, whereas regurgitation (incompetence or reflux) is a failure of preventing the backflow of blood. Both conditions can coexist in the same valve (e.g. aortic stenosis and regurgitation after rheumatic fever).

Valvular disease can be caused by direct leaflet damage or by valve ring damage, or it may be secondary to damage of the papillary muscles or chordae. Major causes of acquired valve disease are as follows:

Drug	Channels						Receptors				Pumps	Clinical effects			Clinical effects		
	Na			Ca	K	I$_f$	α	β	M$_2$	A$_1$	Na$^+$/K$^+$ ATPase	left ventricular function	sinus rate	extra-cardiac	PR interval	QRS width	JT interval
	fast	med	slow														
Lidocaine	□											→	→	□			↓
Mexiletine	□											→	→	□			↓
Tocainide	□											→	→	■			↓
Moricizine	⊗											↓	→	□		↑	
Procainamide		⊘			▨							↓	→	■	↑	↑	↑
Disopyramide		⊘			▨				□			↓	→	▨	↑↓	↑	↑
Quinidine		⊘			▨		□		□			→	↑	▨	↑↓	↑	↑
Propafenone		⊘						▨				↓	↓	▨	↑	↑	
Flecainide			⊘	□								↓	→	□	↑	↑	
Encainide			⊘									↓	→	□	↑	↑	
Bepridil	□			■	▨							↓		□			↑
Verapamil	□			■			▨					↓	↓	□	↑		
Diltiazem	□			▨								↓	↓	□	↑		
Bretylium				■			◐	◐				→	↓	□			↑
Sotalol					■			■				↓	↓	□	↑		↑
Amiodarone	□			□	▨		▨	□				→	↓	■	↑		↑
Alinidine					▨	■								■			
Nadolol								■				↓	↓	□	↑		
Propranolol	□							■				↓	↓	□	↑		
Atropine									■			→	↑	□	↓		
Adenosine										○		↓		□	↑		
Digoxin									○		■	↑	↓	■	↑		↓

relative potency of block: □ low ▨ moderate ■ high
○ = agonist ◐ = agonist/antagonist
⊘ = activated state blocker
⊗ = inactivated state blocker

Fig. 5.14 Spreadsheet approach to the classification of drugs. (A$_1$, adenosine receptor; I$_f$, inward background depolarizing current of pacemaker caused by Na$^+$ and Ca^{2+}, termed 'funny'; M$_2$, muscarinic receptor; Lidocaine, lignocaine.) (Reproduced from *Eur Heart J*. Vol 17, March 1996. Courtesy of WB Saunders Co. Ltd.)

- Mitral stenosis—can be caused by rheumatic fever.
- Mitral regurgitation—can be caused by rheumatic fever, mitral valve prolapse, papillary muscle dysfunction, or valve ring dilatation.
- Aortic stenosis—can be caused by rheumatic fever or calcific degeneration.
- Aortic regurgitation—can be caused by rheumatic fever, aortic dilatation, or rheumatological disorders.

Degenerative valve disease
Degenerative calcific aortic stenosis

Degenerative calcific aortic stenosis accounts for 90% of acquired aortic stenosis. This is an age-related degeneration, more common in the very old (aged over 70 years). Congenital bicuspid aortic valves (usually the valves are tricuspid) occur in 1% of the population. These valves become calcified much earlier in life (from about 50 years of age).

Rigid calcified deposits occur on the sinuses of Valsalva, resulting in thick, immobile valve cusps with narrowing of the orifice. Left ventricular hypertrophy usually results. Intervention is required if angina, syncope, or heart failure result.

Mitral annular calcification

Mitral annular calcification produces mitral regurgitation because the valve ring does not contract properly during systole. The condition also causes mitral stenosis because the bulky deposits prevent opening of the valves. Mitral annular calcification occurs more commonly in the elderly. Mitral stenosis increases the risk of thrombosis within the left atrium with subsequent systemic thromboembolism.

Calcific deposits may interfere with the conduction pathway, leading to arrhythmias, and they may also be a focus for infective endocarditis.

Myxomatous degeneration of the mitral valve (mitral valve prolapse)

Myxomatous degeneration causes billowing or prolapse of the mitral valve during systole, leading to regurgitation. The condition occurs in 15% of patients aged over 70 years. Cusps are thickened because of myxomatous (mucoid) deposition and fibrosis. Usually, this condition is asymptomatic except for a midsystolic click; an audible late systolic murmur indicates regurgitation. In severe disease, the chordae tendineae can rupture causing sudden, severe regurgitation.

Rheumatic heart disease

Rheumatic heart disease is a consequence of rheumatic fever that may have occurred many years previously. The acute process can leave the valves scarred and deformed, causing chronic rheumatic heart disease. This occurs if the onset of acute rheumatic fever is in early childhood and severe, or in chronic rheumatic fever.

Acute rheumatic fever

Acute rheumatic fever is an inflammatory disease caused by an autoimmune reaction initiated by infection with group A streptococci, usually in the throat. It mostly affects children aged 5–15 years. Now rare in the UK (occurring in 0.01% of children), it is common in the Middle East, Eastern Europe, Far East, and South America.

It affects the heart, skin, joints, and central nervous system. Jones's criteria for diagnosis include:

- Carditis involving all three layers (pancarditis).
- Sydenham's chorea (St Vitus dance; rapid, involuntary purposeless movements).
- Polyarthritis affecting the large joints.
- Erythema marginatum (macular rash with erythematous edge).
- Subcutaneous nodules.

Fever, arthralgia, and leucocytosis also commonly occur.

Carditis consists of granulomatous lesions with a central necrotic area (Aschoff nodule). Initially, there are macrophages, lymphocytes, and plasma cells, but these are replaced by fibrous scar tissue. On the valve, Aschoff nodules give rise to small vegetations (verrucae) of platelets and fibrin, which look like beads. Commonly, this affects the mitral valve (65%) or the mitral and aortic valves (25%). Recurrence is common if persistent carditis is present.

Chronic rheumatic fever

Chronic rheumatic fever is repeated attacks of rheumatic fever leading to chronic rheumatic heart disease, occurring in over half the patients with rheumatic carditis. This leads to commissural fusion, shortening/thickening of the chordae, and cusp fibrosis—the so-called fish-mouth or button-hole mitral valve deformity. Secondary changes in the heart occur as a result of:

- Mitral stenosis and regurgitation—leads to left atrial hypertrophy, pulmonary hypertension, atrial fibrillation, and thrombosis.
- Aortic stenosis—leads to left ventricular hypertrophy and arrhythmia.
- Aortic regurgitation—leads to left ventricular hypertrophy and dilatation.

Infective endocarditis

Infective endocarditis is an infection of the endocardium or vascular endothelium, usually involving the heart valves. In the past, it was classified as acute or subacute (Fig. 5.15); now it is classified according to the causative organism. The incidence is 6–7 per 100 000 in the UK, but it is more common in developing countries.

Infective endocarditis occurs more commonly on valves that have been previously damaged or are congenitally abnormal. Inflammation of the valve causes destruction and scarring.

Vegetations (consisting of fibrin, platelets, and the infecting organism) usually arise on the valves.

Acute compared with subacute manifestations of infective endocarditis		
Features	Acute	Subacute
Virulence of organism	High	Moderate or low
State of valve before infection	Normal	Injured or abnormal
Type of infection	Necrotizing and invasive	Less destructive
Macroscopic vegetations	Larger and may cause emboli	Small to large
Presentation	Fever, rigors, malaise, splenomegaly, heart murmur	Low-grade fever, weight loss, flu-like syndrome, heart murmur
Course	Death occurs in 50% within days	Protracted course; often less fatal

Fig. 5.15 Acute compared with subacute manifestations of infective endocarditis.

Causative agents include:
- *Streptococcus viridans*—subacute; common after dental procedures, tonsillectomy, or bronchoscopy.
- *Staphylococcus aureus*—acute; common in patients with indwelling catheters.
- *Enterococcus faecalis*—common in patients with pelvic infections or after having pelvic surgery.
- *Coxiella burnetti* (Q fever)—subacute.
- *Staphylococcus epidermidis, Aspergillus, Candida, Brucella, Histoplasma*—common in drug addicts and patients with prosthetic heart valves.

Sequelae of infective endocarditis include:
- Acute valve incompetence.
- Emboli to spleen, kidneys, and brain.
- Glomerulonephritis and renal failure.

Non-bacterial thrombotic (marantic) endocarditis
Marantic endocarditis causes small sterile fibrin and platelet thrombi on valves (mostly mitral) along the lines of closure. There is no inflammation or valvular damage. It usually occurs in cancer or a prolonged debilitating illness, and it is caused by a hypercoagulable state.

Endocarditis of systemic lupus erythematosus (Libman–Sacks disease)
Mitral and tricuspid valves are most commonly affected by Libman–Sacks disease. Fibrinoid necrosis, mucoid degeneration, and small vegetations on either side of the cusps may develop. Healing of vegetations may cause valve deformity.

Carcinoid heart disease
Argentaffinomas (tumours of the argentaffin cells of the intestine) produce physiologically active substances (e.g. 5-hydroxytryptamine (serotonin), bradykinin, prostaglandins), which cause thickening of the tricuspid and pulmonary valve and parts of the right ventricle. The left side is usually unaffected.

Diseases of the myocardium

Myocardial disease can be categorized as either a cardiomyopathy or a specific heart muscle disease:
- A cardiomyopathy is any chronic disease affecting the muscle of the heart for which the cause is unknown (i.e. idiopathic, primary).
- Specific heart muscle disease is a heart muscle disease for which the cause is known or associated with other disorders.

Myocardial dysfunction may also be a result of:
- Congenital heart disease.
- Hypertension.
- Ischaemia.
- Valve disease.
- Pericardial disease.

Myocarditis is inflammation of the myocardium, and it is one of the main functional classes of specific heart muscle disease.

Cardiomyopathy
Cardiomyopathy is often functionally classified according to presentation into the following diseases:

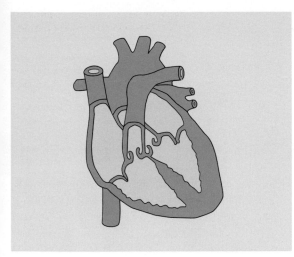

Fig. 5.16 A normal heart for comparison with the cardiomyopathic hearts shown in Figs 5.17–5.19.

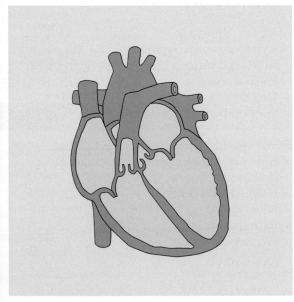

Fig. 5.17 Dilated cardiomyopathy. The ventricles are thin and dilated. Compare with Fig. 5.16.

- Dilated (congestive) cardiomyopathy (85%)—with dilated left ventricle and impaired systolic function.
- Hypertrophic (obstructive) cardiomyopathy (10%)—hypertrophy of ventricles, especially the interventricular septum; reduced diastolic filling.
- Restrictive cardiomyopathy (5%)—decreased ventricular compliance restricts ventricular filling.

Dilated cardiomyopathy

Dilated cardiomyopathy (Figs 5.16 and 5.17) causes dilated ventricles and poor contraction. Its prevalence is 0.2%.

Pathogenic factors include:
- Genetic defect.
- Alcohol toxicity.
- Postviral myocarditis—some myocarditis progresses to ventricular dilatation.
- Peripartum—may be caused by physiological, pathological, or metabolic changes in pregnancy.

Other associations include:
- Cardiovascular disease (e.g. ischaemia, hypertension).
- Systemic disease (e.g. sarcoidosis, systemic lupus erythematosus, haemochromatosis).
- Neuromuscular disease (e.g. muscular dystrophy, Friedreich's ataxia).
- Haemochromatosis.
- Glycogen storage disorder.
- Primary heart muscle disease (e.g. amyloidosis).
- Drug therapy: cytotoxic drugs (e.g. cyclophosphamide).

The morphology of dilated cardiomyopathy is as follows:
- Cardiomegaly (up to 900 g), but dilated thin walls in all chambers.
- Irregular myocyte hypertrophy and fibrosis.

Dilated cardiomyopathy can cause heart failure, arrhythmia, and emboli. Investigations include chest radiography, electrocardiography, and cardiac biopsy. Mortality is 40% within 2 years.

Hypertrophic (obstructive) cardiomyopathy

Hypertrophic cardiomyopathy (HCM) (Fig. 5.18) is characterized by hypertrophy of the ventricles and septum; often it is asymmetrical. The disease causes distorted contraction and abnormal mitral valve movement. It is more common in young adults, and 50% of cases are inherited (autosomal dominant). The morphology of the hypertrophic cardiomyopathy is as follows:
- Asymmetrical septal hypertrophy.
- Left ventricular cavity is banana-like.
- Myofibre hypertrophy and disarray.
- Patchy fibrosis.

Hypertrophic cardiomyopathy can also cause dyspnoea, angina, syncope, and sudden death.

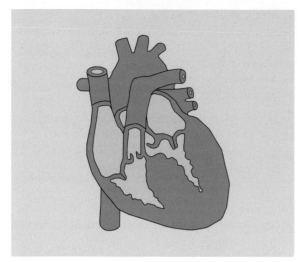

Fig. 5.18 Hypertrophic cardiomyopathy. There is an increase in ventricular mass. Compare with Fig. 5.16.

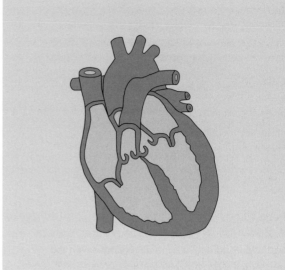

Fig. 5.19 Restrictive cardiomyopathy. The heart is of normal size, but the ventricles are stiff. Compare with Fig. 5.16.

Characteristic findings include a fourth heart sound, jerky pulse, and systolic murmur. The course of the disease is very variable; most patients are unchanged for years.

Restrictive cardiomyopathy

Restrictive cardiomyopathy (Fig. 5.19) is a stiffening of the endomyocardium with restricted ventricular filling. It is often associated with:

- Amyloidosis—most common form in the UK.
- Endomyocardial fibrosis—children and young adults in Africa.
- Loeffler's endocarditis—found in temperate climates.

There is interstitial myocardial fibrosis (associated with eosinophilia in the latter two conditions). Dyspnoea, fatigue, and emboli may be the presenting features. Symptoms are often similar to those seen in constrictive pericarditis.

Specific heart muscle disease
Myocarditis

Myocarditis is inflammation of the myocardium. Causes include:

- Infection—viruses (coxsackievirus, influenza, rubella, echovirus, polio); bacteria (*Corynebacterium*—diphtheria, *Rickettsia*, *Chlamydia*); protozoa (*Trypanosoma cruzi*—Chagas' disease, *Toxoplasma gondii*); fungi (*Candida*).
- Immune-mediated reactions—after infections (viral or rheumatic fever); systemic lupus erythematosus; transplant rejection; chemicals, radiation, and drugs (chloroquine, methyldopa, lead poisoning).
- Idiopathic causes—sarcoidosis, giant cell myocarditis.

The morphology of myocarditis is as follows:

- Flabby myocardium with dilatation in all four chambers.
- Haemorrhagic mottling.
- Mural thrombi.
- Inflammatory infiltrate with focal myocyte necrosis and fibrosis.

Patients present with fever, dyspnoea, angina, arrhythmia, and heart failure; the presentation is similar to myocardial infarction.

Other diseases

Other specific heart muscle diseases are generally associated with cardiotoxic agents, which cause myocyte swelling, fatty change, and lysis.

Fibrosis and scarring usually replace the focal lesions.

The various causes are explained below.

Alcohol

Alcohol causes a similar morphology to dilated cardiomyopathy. It may be associated with thiamine deficiency.

Adriamycin (doxorubicin) and other drugs

These cytotoxic drugs in toxic levels cause oxidation of the myocyte membranes, causing a similar morphology to dilated cardiomyopathy.

Catecholamines

Either exogenous (e.g. administered adrenaline) or endogenous (e.g. in phaeochromocytoma) catecholamines can cause tachycardia and vasoconstriction, leading to patchy ischaemic necrosis. This leads to a dilated cardiomyopathy. Cocaine may have a similar effect as it stops noradrenaline uptake.

Peripartum state

A dilated heart is found several months before and after delivery. The mechanism for this is uncertain, but it may include hypertension, volume overload, nutritional deficiency, immune reaction, or metabolic dysfunction. In 50% of these patients, function is restored several months later.

Amyloidosis

Amyloidosis may be systemic or isolated. It may produce arrhythmia or restrictive cardiomyopathy.

Iron overload

Patients with iron overload present with a dilated cardiomyopathy. This is often found in hereditary haemochromatosis and haemosiderosis (excess blood transfusion).

Diseases of the pericardium

Fluid accumulation in the pericardial sac

Normally, the pericardial sac contains 50 mL of serous fluid. Its functions include:

- Lubrication.
- Prevention of sudden deformation or dislocation.
- A barrier to the spread of infection.

Slow effusions allow greater volumes to accumulate before reaching the clinical threshold.

Pericardial effusion

A pericardial effusion:

- Is an accumulation of fluid in the pericardial cavity.
- Can be caused by any condition causing pericarditis.
- Can usually be morphologically classified as serous, serosanguineous, or chylous.

The effusion collects in the closed cavity and causes distension. When the pericardium cannot distend any more, pressure builds up and cardiac tamponade results (impaired ventricular filling leading to loss of cardiac output).

Serous

In a serous effusion, there is a smooth glistening serosa. Fluid accumulates slowly. The effusion is caused by heart failure and hypoproteinaemia.

Serosanguineous

These effusions are caused by blunt chest trauma.

Chylous

Chylous effusions are caused by lymphatic obstruction.

Haemopericardium

Haemopericardium is the accumulation of blood in the pericardial sac. It is caused by:

- Myocardial rupture after a myocardial infarction.
- Rupture of the intrapericardial aorta.
- Haemorrhage from an abscess or tumour.
- Trauma.

If the accumulation of blood is greater than 200–300 mL, cardiac tamponade can result. Cardiac tamponade occurs when there is an abnormal external pressure on the heart. This impairs ventricular filling and affects cardiac output.

Clinical features of cardiac tamponade are of heart failure, including a raised jugular venous pressure, Kussmaul's sign, exaggerated pulsus paradoxus, soft heart sounds, and the apex beat may not be palpable. If a frictional rub was present, it may be quieter than before as the fluid separates the parietal and visceral pericardium.

An echocardiogram is the best method for diagnosing a pericardial effusion.

Cardiac tamponade is one of the causes of electromechanical dissociation. This is when the ventricular contraction is independent of the electrical activity of the heart. That is, the electrical signal to contract is being sent to the ventricles, but no organized contraction occurs, and cardiac arrest results.

Other causes of electromechanical dissociation include:

- Tension pneumothorax.
- Hypovolaemia.

- Massive pulmonary embolism.
- Drug overdose.
- Hypothermia.

Electromechanical dissociation is an acute cardiorespiratory arrest, and it needs immediate treatment.

The effusion must be tapped (pericardiocentesis) if it severely compromises the circulation (i.e. when the effusion develops rapidly).

Reaccumulation occurs with purulent, tuberculous, and malignant effusions.

Pericarditis

Pericarditis is an inflammation of the pericardium leading to sharp substernal chest pain that radiates to the back, and that is aggravated by movement and respiration. Common causes are listed in Fig. 5.20.

Acute pericarditis

Commonly, acute pericarditis is caused by an acute viral (coxsackievirus) infection or a myocardial infarction. Morphologically acute pericarditis can be separated into:

- Serous—slowly accumulating serous exudate with inflammatory cells.
- Fibrinous/serofibrinous—most common, may resolve completely or leave adhesions.

Common causes of pericarditis	
Cause	**Pathology**
Viral (coxsackievirus)	Fibrinous
Myocardial infarction	Fibrinous and may lead to fibrous adhesions
Uraemia	Fibrinous
Carcinoma (metastatic spread, often from the lung)	Serous or haemorrhagic
Connective tissue disease (rheumatic fever)	Fibrinous
Bacterial	Purulent
Tuberculosis	Caseous
After cardiac surgery	Fibrinous
Dressler's syndrome (after a myocardial infarction)	Autoimmune

Fig. 5.20 Common causes of pericarditis.

- Suppurative (purulent)—bacterial/fungal infection with pus; may produce constrictive pericarditis.
- Haemorrhagic—blood exudate with fibrin or pus; may calcify.
- Caseous—leads to constrictive pericarditis; caused by tuberculosis.

Chronic pericarditis
Healing of pericarditis can result in complete resolution, thick plaques, or adhesions.

Adhesive pericarditis
In adhesive pericarditis, the parietal pericardium becomes attached to the mediastinum and the pericardial sac no longer exists. The heart dilates and hypertrophies.

Constrictive pericarditis
In constrictive pericarditis, there is a thick, fibrous, often calcified pericardial sac that encases the heart, limiting cardiac filling and reducing cardiac output. Symptoms of heart failure result.

Rheumatic disease of the pericardium
Pericarditis occurs in 30% of people with severe chronic rheumatoid arthritis. Granulomas may lead to fibrous adhesions, causing constrictive pericarditis.

Inflammatory vascular disease

Concepts and classification
The vasculitides are a group of conditions characterized by vasculitis (inflammation and damage of the vessel walls) (Fig. 5.21). They may be classified by pathogenesis (infective, immune-mediated, or idiopathic) or by the size of the vessel affected (large, medium, or small).

Most systemic vasculitides probably involve an immunological process. Many different processes have been described. There may be deposition of circulating antigen–antibody complexes in conditions such as systemic lupus erythematosus. Antibodies may react with fixed tissue antigens as in Kawasaki syndrome. Temporal arteritis involves delayed-type hypersensitivity reactions with granuloma formation.

The presence of anti-neutrophilic cytoplasmic autoantibodies (ANCA), which react with antigens in the cytoplasm of neutrophils, can be seen in

Vessels affected by vasculitides		
Vessel size	Arteries	Disease
Large/ medium	Aorta Carotid Temporal	Giant cell arteritis, Takayasu's arteritis
Medium/ small	Coronary Mesenteric	Polyarteritis nodosa, Kawasaki disease
Small/ arteriole	Glomeruli and arterioles	Wegener's granulomatosis, microscopic polyarteritis nodosa
Arteriole/ capillary	—	Henoch–Schönlein purpura, Cutaneous leucocytoclastic
Veins	—	Buerger's disease

Fig. 5.21 Vessels affected by vasculitides.

many vasculitides. The antigen may be perinuclear (p-ANCA) or cytoplasmic (c-ANCA).

Infectious vasculitides
The causes of infectious vasculitides may be:
- Bacterial (e.g. *Neisseria*).
- Viral causes (e.g. herpes).
- Other infectious causes such as *Rickettsia* (Rocky Mountain spotted fever), spirochaetes (syphilis), or fungi (*Aspergillus*).

Immunological vasculitides
The immunological vasculitides can be classified as:
- Immune-complex—Henoch–Schönlein purpura, systemic lupus erythematosus.
- Direct antibody—Goodpasture's syndrome (anti-basement membrane antibodies), Kawasaki disease.
- ANCA-associated—Wegener's granulomatosis, microscopic polyarteritis.
- Cell-mediated—organ rejection.

Idiopathic vasculitides
Giant-cell (temporal) arteritis
Giant-cell arteritis is the most common of the vasculitides, occurring in the elderly and being rare in those younger than 55 years of age. There is focal granulomatous inflammation of medium and small arteries, especially the cranial vessels. It usually presents with headache and facial pain and polymyalgia rheumatica (flu-like aches and fever). The erythrocyte sedimentation ratio (ESR) and/or C reactive protein (CRP) are usually raised. Visual disturbances develop in about half affected individuals and may lead to blindness without

prompt intervention. Diagnosis is by temporal artery biopsy; microscopically, the following signs are seen:
- Granulations with giant cells.
- General leucocytic infiltrate.
- Fibrosis of the intima and stenosis.

There is often associated thrombosis. Diagnosis is by biopsy, which may be negative in one third of cases. Treatment is with corticosteroids.

Takayasu's disease (aortic arch syndrome)
Takayasu's disease typically affects females in the 20–40-year-old age group. It is most common in Asia. It is a granulomatous vasculitis of medium-to-large arteries, especially the aorta and the great vessels. Patients present with visual disturbances, neurological deficits, and diminished upper pulses ('pulseless disease'). If the renal arteries are involved, hypertension may result. There is thickening of the aortic wall with mononuclear cell infiltrates. Fibrosis and granulomas may result.

Polyarteritis nodosa
Polyarteritis nodosa is twice as common in males than in females, usually occurring in the middle aged. It is associated with the hepatitis B surface (s) antigen. p-ANCA may have a role.

Fibrinoid necrosis of medium-to-small arteries occurs, especially of the main viscera (e.g. coronary, renal, and hepatic arteries). The pulmonary arteries are not usually affected. Presenting features can be general (e.g. fever) or relate to the system involved:
- Renal—hypertension, renal failure.
- Cardiac—myocardial infarction, heart failure.
- Central nervous system—hemiplegia, psychoses.
- Gastrointestinal—abdominal pain, melaena.

Segmental lesions occur, with fibrinoid necrosis of the wall and a neutrophil infiltrate. Healing results in thickening and aneurysmal dilatation. A type of polyarteritis nodosa known as Churg–Strauss syndrome affects the lungs. Diagnosis is by biopsy; treatment is with anti-viral therapy for hepatitis B associated polyarteritis or immunosuppression.

Kawasaki syndrome (mucocutaneous lymph node syndrome)
Kawasaki syndrome is an acute febrile illness of young children. Patients present with lymphadenopathy, rash, erythema, peeling skin, and (in 20% of those affected) coronary arteritis with

aneurysms, which may lead to myocardial infarction or sudden cardiac death.

Similar lesions occur to those seen in polyarteritis nodosa. Aspirin and γ-globulin therapy is thought to prevent cardiac complications.

Microscopic polyarteritis (leucocytoclastic angiitis)

Microscopic polyarteritis is a fibrinoid necrosis of the smallest vessels, and it is thought to be a form of hypersensitivity reaction. Typically, there is an acute onset with a precipitating agent (e.g. bacteria) and involvement of the skin or viscera. There may be little neutrophilic infiltrate.

Wegener's granulomatosis

The majority of cases are in patients aged over 50 years. The condition consists of a triad of symptoms:

- Necrotizing vasculitis of the lung and upper respiratory tract.
- Granulomas of the respiratory tract.
- Glomerulonephritis of the kidneys.

c-ANCA type autoantibodies are usually present. Lesions are similar to those of polyarteritis nodosa, but granulomas also occur. Treatment is by immunosuppression (using prednisolone and cyclophosphamide).

Thromboangiitis obliterans (Buerger's disease)

Thromboangiitis obliterans is typically found in male smokers aged under 35 years. It is twice as common in Jews than in non-Jews. It involves inflammation of the vessels of the lower limbs. Nodular phlebitis (inflammation of veins) and ischaemia of the extremities results. There is neutrophilic infiltration with thrombi and giant-cell formation.

Frequently, the condition is painful and leads to gangrene if smoking is not stopped.

Vasculitis in systemic disease

Many diseases have vasculitis as a component.

Systemic lupus erythematosus

Systemic lupus erythematosus (SLE) affects capillaries, arterioles, and venules. An inflammatory vasculitis is predominant; neutrophils are more common than lymphocytes. Vasculitic lesions on the skin, muscle, and brain are common. Raynaud's phenomenon may also be present. A similar pathology exists in other connective tissue disorders (e.g. scleroderma, cryoglobulinaemia).

Henoch–Schönlein purpura

This is a hypersensitivity reaction that is often preceded by infection. Purpuric rashes caused by inflammation of capillaries and venules are present on the legs and buttocks. Abdominal pain, arthritis, haematuria, and nephritis may also occur.

Rheumatoid vasculitis

Vasculitis is one of the extra-articular features of rheumatoid arthritis.

Infectious vasculitis

Systemic infections can result in a vasculitis. These often produce a purpuric rash due to a hypersensitivity reaction.

Raynaud's disease

Raynaud's disease is not strictly a vasculitis, but it is worth considering here as it has some features in common with those of other vasculitides.

Raynaud's disease affects 5% of the population, and it is mainly found in young healthy women. There is pallor and cyanosis caused by vasospasm of the small arteries/arterioles in the hands and feet. The exact aetiology is unknown, but it is thought to be due to increased vasomotor responses to cold or emotion.

Raynaud's phenomenon refers to the decrease in blood flow that occurs secondary to the narrowing of the arteries that supply the extremities. It implies a known aetiology; this can be atherosclerosis, systemic lupus erythematosus, scleroderma, or Buerger's disease.

Congenital abnormalities of the heart

Congenital heart defects have an incidence of 6–8 per 1000 liveborn infants. They may present in the first year of life or remain asymptomatic for life.

Left-to-right shunts

Left-to-right shunts very rarely cause cyanosis.

Atrial septal defect

An atrial septal defect (ASD) is caused by a failure of proper closure of the foramen ovale or by a defect in the septum secundum, see p. 13 (Fig. 5.22). Blood moves from the left atrium into the right atrium because of the pressure difference. Atrial septal defects make up 10% of all congenital heart defects.

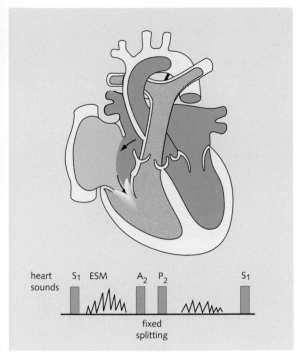

heart
sounds   S₁ ESM   A₂ P₂   S₁

fixed
splitting

Fig. 5.22 Atrial septal defect. (S_1, first heart sound from closure of mitral and tricuspid valves; A_2, heart sound from closure of aortic valve; ESM, ejection systolic murmur; P_2, heart sound from closure of pulmonary valve.) (Courtesy of Lissauer and Clayden, 2001.)

Frequently, the child is asymptomatic, but clinical features can include:
- Recurrent chest infections, heart failure, and arrhythmias.
- Fixed, widely split second heart sound.
- Ejection systolic murmur, best heard in the third intercostal space, produced by increased flow across the pulmonary valve (left-to-right shunt).

Electrocardiography, chest radiography, and echocardiography will confirm the diagnosis. In children with symptoms, treatment is by a catheter-delivered device or surgery.

Ventricular septal defect

A ventricular septal defect (VSD) is a failure of fusion of the interventricular septum or endocardial cushions, see p.13 (Fig. 5.23). Blood shunts through a hole in the interventricular septum.

Ventricular septal defects make up 30% of all congenital heart lesions. The patient may be asymptomatic, but clinical features can include:
- Heart failure, failure to thrive, recurrent chest infections.
- Palpable parasternal thrill.

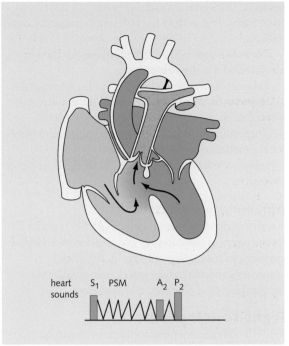

heart
sounds   S₁ PSM   A₂ P₂

Fig. 5.23 Ventricular septal defect. (S_1, first heart sound from closure of mitral and tricuspid valves; A_2, heart sound from closure of aortic valve; PSM, pansystolic murmur; P_2, heart sound from closure of pulmonary valve.) (Courtesy of Lissauer and Clayden, 2001.)

- Loud pansystolic murmur at lower left sternal edge.

Electrocardiography, echocardiography, and chest radiography will confirm the diagnosis.

Most ventricular septal defects will close spontaneously within the first 2 years of life. However, 10% will require drug therapy (for heart failure) or surgery.

If there is a large left-to-right shunt, there will be a great deal of blood entering the right ventricle and pulmonary circulation, causing pulmonary hypertension. Eventually, the pulmonary hypertension will cause irreversible damage to the pulmonary vasculature. This will cause right ventricular hypertrophy, which may eventually lead to reversal of the shunt from right to left. This is Eisenmenger's syndrome and it often leads to cyanosis (Fig. 5.24).

Other large left-to-right shunts (e.g. atrial septal defects or patent ductus arteriosus) can also lead to Eisenmenger's syndrome.

Patent ductus arteriosus

Patent ductus arteriosus is caused by an open ductus arteriosus, which allows the communication of blood between the systemic and pulmonary circulations (Fig. 5.25). It accounts for 10% of all congenital heart defects.

There is a continuous murmur beneath the left clavicle and a collapsing pulse.

Echocardiography is the most useful investigation.

In preterm infants, the duct will ultimately close, but it can be closed with indometacin (inhibits prostaglandin production), or it may require closure with a catheter-delivered device.

Infective endocarditis may result if the duct never closes.

Atrioventricular septal defect

An atrioventricular septal defect (AVSD) results from failure of the superior and inferior endocardial cushions to fuse, see p. 13 (Fig. 5.26). This is commonly seen in babies with Down syndrome. Surgical repair is complex and hazardous.

Right-to-left shunts

Right-to-left shunts commonly cause cyanosis.

Tetralogy of Fallot

Tetralogy of Fallot (Fig. 5.27) is a combination of:
- Large ventricular septal defect.
- Pulmonary stenosis.
- Right ventricular hypertrophy.
- Aorta overriding the interventricular septum.

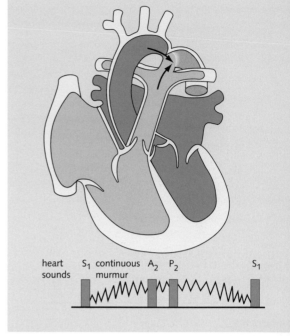

Fig. 5.25 Patent ductus arteriosus. This is often found with coarctation of the aorta (shown). It allows mixing of systemic and pulmonary blood. Movement of blood within the ductus can occur in both directions depending upon the relative pressures in the aorta and the pulmonary trunk. (S_1, first heart sound from closure of mitral and tricuspid valves; A_2, heart sound from closure of aortic valve; P_2, heart sound from closure of pulmonary valve.) (Courtesy of Lissauer and Clayden, 1997.)

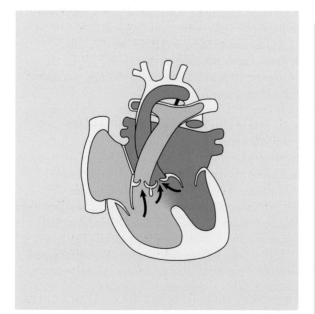

Fig. 5.24 Eisenmenger's syndrome. The shunt has reversed (and now goes from right to left). Less blood now goes into the pulmonary trunk and the patient becomes cyanosed. (Courtesy of Lissauer and Clayden, 2001.)

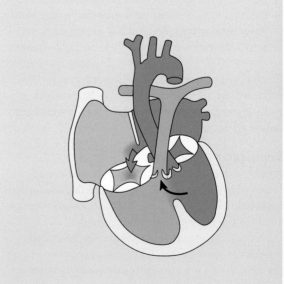

Fig. 5.26 Atrioventricular septal defect (AVSD). There is very little separation between the atria and ventricles. (Courtesy of Lissauer and Clayden, 2001.)

The tetralogy occurs in 6% of children with heart defects. Severe cyanosis with hypercyanotic episodes may result. A loud ejection systolic murmur is heard in the third left intercostal space, and finger clubbing may develop. Corrective surgery is required, which can be started at 4–6 months of age.

Transposition of the great arteries

Transposition of the great arteries occurs when the truncoconal septum develops, but it does not spiral (Fig. 5.28). The left ventricle pumps blood into the pulmonary trunk and the right ventricle pumps blood into the aorta. There is usually also an atrial septal defect, ventricular septal defect, or patent ductus arteriosus to allow blood to mix, otherwise this would be incompatible with life.

Transposition of the great arteries occurs in 4% of cardiac defects. Severe cyanosis may result. There may be finger clubbing and various murmurs. Ultimately surgical treatment is required.

Persistent truncus arteriosus

The truncoconal septum fails to form, leading to a common outflow tract for both ventricles. There is also a ventricular septal defect in this very rare condition.

Tricuspid atresia

In tricuspid atresia, there is an absence of the tricuspid valve, causing poor pulmonary circulation. The neonate has a duct-dependent circulation (i.e. other communications are needed between the arterial and venous systems to prevent serious cyanosis). Surgery is required to replace the tricuspid valve.

Obstructive congenital defects
Coarctation of the aorta

Coarctation of the aorta is a narrowing of the aorta around the area of the ductus arteriosus (Fig. 5.29). It is frequently associated with a ventricular septal defect and a bicuspid aortic valve. Coarctation occurs in 7% of children with congenital heart defects. The diagnosis can be made from weak or absent femoral pulses. There is also an ejection systolic murmur heard at the back. Surgery is required.

Pulmonary stenosis with intact interventricular septum

Of those children with heart defects, 7% present with a stenosis of the pulmonary valve (Fig. 5.30); most are asymptomatic. An ejection systolic murmur

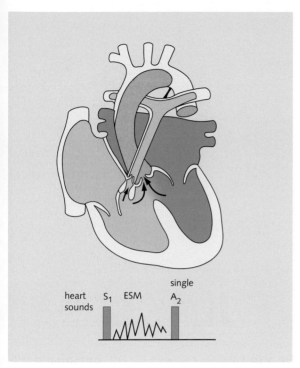

Fig. 5.27 Tetralogy of Fallot. The right-to-left shunt that results causes cyanosis. (S₁, first heart sound from closure of mitral and tricuspid valves; A₂, heart sound from closure of aortic valve; ESM, ejection systolic murmur.) (Courtesy of Lissauer and Clayden, 2001.)

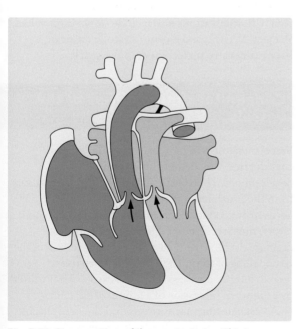

Fig. 5.28 Transposition of the great arteries. This is incompatible with life without a ventricular (VSD) or atrial septal defect (ASD) or a patent ductus arteriosus. (Courtesy of Lissauer and Clayden, 2001.)

Link the problems that can occur in embryological development with the pressure changes that occur in the cardiac cycle to work out what sort of shunting mechanism occurs with each defect. Also, any shunt that occurs is going to cause turbulent flow, so the timing of the shunt in the cardiac cycle will tell you what type of murmur occurs. For example, a ventricular septal defect is a defect in the development of the interventricular septum. The left ventricular pressure is greater than the right because of its larger muscle mass, so, therefore, blood is going to flow from left to right. As this shunt occurs throughout systole a pansystolic murmur occurs.

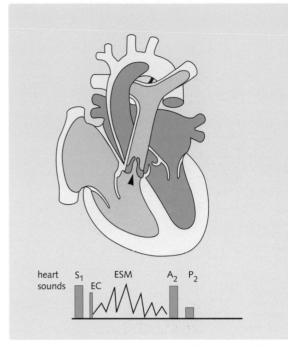

Fig. 5.30 Pulmonary stenosis. (S_1, first heart sound from closure of mitral and tricuspid valves; A_2, heart sound from closure of aortic valve; EC, ejection click; ESM, ejection systolic murmur; P_2, heart sound from closure of pulmonary valve.) (Courtesy of Lissauer and Clayden, 2001.)

and ejection click may be heard. Treatment is indicated when right ventricular hypertrophy occurs or the stenosis worsens.

Aortic stenosis

Stenosis of the aortic valve occurs in 6% of neonates with heart defects (Fig. 5.31). Usually there is

associated mitral stenosis and coarctation of the aorta. There may be heart failure, syncope, and chest pain. Clinical features also include slow-rising pulses, an ejection click, and ejection systolic murmur. Eventually valve replacement is necessary.

Congenital abnormalities of the vessels

Vascular anatomy is complex, and it undergoes considerable remodelling during embryological development. There are many areas where departures from the usual development can occur. These do not necessarily produce deficiencies in the flow of blood; rather, most represent an alternative supply and drainage of the same tissue. For example, errors in the remodelling of the great vessels may give rise to double inferior and superior venae cavae: this is caused by a failure of regression of a primitive element.

A vascular ring may form around the oesophagus and trachea, causing difficulty in swallowing and breathing. This is caused by a persistent right dorsal aorta or it may result from other problems in aortic arch development.

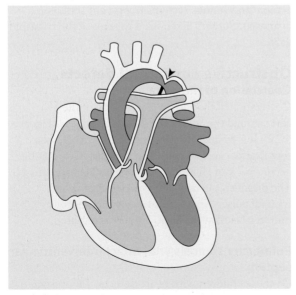

Fig. 5.29 Coarctation of the aorta, causing stenosis. (Courtesy of Lissauer and Clayden, 2001.)

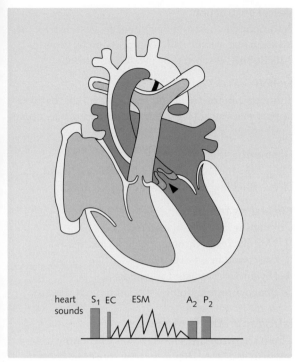

Fig. 5.31 Aortic stenosis. (S_1, first heart sound from closure of mitral and tricuspid valves; A_2, heart sound from closure of aortic valve; EC, ejection click; ESM, ejection systolic murmur; P_2, heart sound from closure of pulmonary valve.) (Courtesy of Lissauer and Clayden, 2001.)

Lymphoedema may result from hypoplasia of the lymphatic system.

Abnormalities in the coronary circulation may sometimes be normal (e.g. when branches of the left coronary artery arise directly from the aorta), or they may lead to ischaemia and infarction of the myocardium.

Furthermore, some abnormalities may be protective. For example, sometimes the kidney has a double renal arterial supply, which will help to maintain renal perfusion in hypovolaemia.

Two important anomalies of the circulation are:
- Arteriovenous fistulae.
- Berry aneurysms.

Arteriovenous fistula

An arteriovenous fistula is an abnormal communication between an artery and a vein. This may be congenital in origin or secondary to trauma, inflammation, or a healed ruptured aneurysm. Fistulae may cause shunting of blood, bypassing circulations and increasing venous return thereby increasing cardiac output. This may predispose to heart failure.

Fistulae may be seen in Paget's disease of the bone, where the increased blood flow through the affected bones may eventually lead to heart failure.

Arteriovenous fistulae are used in haemodialysis for renal patients. Artificial arteriovenous fistulae can be surgically placed between the radial artery and cephalic vein. This causes the vein to distend and thicken, enabling large bore needles to be inserted. These take blood to and from the dialysis machine.

Berry aneurysm

Berry aneurysms are found in about 2% of post mortem examinations, and they are the most common intracranial aneurysm. They are small saccular aneurysms in the cerebral vessels. They can measure about 0.2–3.0 cm in diameter, but are usually around 1.0 cm. They frequently occur at branch points in the circle of Willis (Fig. 5.32). These aneurysms are commonly seen in patients with coarctation of the aorta and polycystic renal disease.

Berry aneurysms are asymptomatic until they rupture (usually when the patient is aged between 40 and 60 years). Rupture is more common in males. Predisposing factors to rupture include smoking, hypertension, and atheroma. The original outpouching is caused by local focal wall weakness. This then gets larger as a result of the haemodynamics in the lumen. Eventually rupture may occur. Rupture of berry aneurysms results in a subarachnoid haemorrhage. This presents with a sudden-onset severe headache, and it may be fatal.

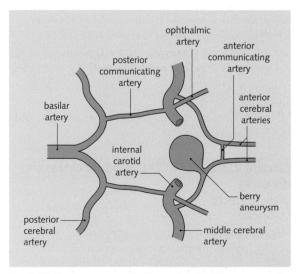

Fig. 5.32 Berry aneurysm in the circle of Willis.

109

Neoplastic heart disease

Primary cardiac tumours
Primary cardiac tumours include myxoma, lipoma, papillary fibroelastoma, rhabdomyoma, and sarcoma. They are extremely rare.

Myxoma
Myxomas account for 25% of primary cardiac tumours. Presentation can be at any age, but mostly it occurs in adults; 75% of myxomas occur in the left atrium. They can be polyploid or pedunculated masses, arising from undifferentiated connective tissue in the subendocardial layer. If pedunculated, the tumour mass may have limited movement within the heart chamber, sufficient to periodically occlude cardiac outflow (ball-valve obstruction). Of patients with myxoma, 50% show signs and symptoms of mitral valve disease. Myxomatous masses can fragment and produce emboli.

Lipoma
Lipomas usually occur in the interatrial septum. They are well circumscribed, poorly encapsulated adipose tissue.

Papillary fibroelastoma
Papillary fibroelastomas are filamentous projections found in right-sided valves in children and left-sided valves in adults. They are composed of connective tissue with smooth muscle and fibroblasts.

Rhabdomyoma
Many rhabdomyomas occur in neonates, causing stillbirth or death in the first few days of life. They are often multiple, and they arise from cardiac muscle. They have strands in the cytoplasm radiating out of the nucleus, and so they are called spider cells.

Sarcoma
Malignant tumours include rhabdomyosarcomas and angiosarcomas.

Cardiovascular effects of neoplastic disease
Direct effects
Metastases
Metastases that develop in the myocardium are usually from bronchial carcinomas or malignant melanomas. They are much more common than primary tumours of cardiac tissue.

Vessel obstruction
A tumour can obstruct neighbouring vessels by local invasion into vessel walls, compression by growth outside the vessel, and by producing emboli.

Emboli
Tumours can fragment and send off emboli that will impact in a vessel (e.g. a tumour in the leg may cause a pulmonary embolus).

Haemorrhage
Malignant tumours on mucosa can ulcerate and bleed. Bleeding can also occur into a tumour.

Circulating factors
Circulating factors can lead to:
- Non-bacterial thrombotic endocarditis.
- Carcinoid heart disease.
- Myeloma-associated amyloidosis.
- Phaeochromocytoma-associated heart disease.

Iatrogenic effects of therapy
There are many unwanted effects of therapy of neoplastic disease. Radiotherapy causes lethargy, appetite loss, and rashes, for example. Chemotherapy causes nausea, vomiting, alopecia, and marrow suppression. Each modality and substance has its own specific side effects. Surgical therapy can be risky and complicated, especially as some tissues are highly vascularized. However, there are few general iatrogenic effects that affect the cardiovascular system.

Neoplastic vascular disease

Benign tumours and related conditions
Haemangioma
Haemangiomas are common, especially in children; they make up approximately 7% of all benign tumours. Haemangiomas are usually subdivided into capillary haemangioma, juvenile capillary haemangioma, cavernous haemangioma, and granuloma pyogenicum.

Capillary haemangioma
Capillary haemangiomas occur mostly in skin and mucous membranes. These are well-defined, encapsulated aggregates of capillaries. They may be thrombosed.

Juvenile capillary ('strawberry') haemangioma
Juvenile capillary haemangiomas are present at birth on the face and scalp of infants. They grow rapidly

for the first few months then regress and disappear by the age of 5 years.

Cavernous haemangioma
Cavernous haemangiomas are large, cavernous, vascular channels that are not encapsulated. They involve skin, mucous membranes, the central nervous system, and the liver.

Granuloma pyogenicum
Granuloma pyogenicum is an ulcerated version of capillary haemangioma, often caused by trauma. Typically, it is composed of capillaries with oedema, inflammatory cells, and granulation tissue. Granuloma gravidum occurs in the gum of up to 5% of pregnant women.

Glomangioma
Glomangiomas are painful tumours of the glomus body (a receptor in the smooth muscle of arteries that is sensitive to temperature; i.e. at arteriovenous anastomoses in the skin). Glomangiomas are usually found in fingers or nail beds. They are branching vascular channels with aggregates of glomus bodies.

Telangiectasia
Telangiectasias are aggregations of prominent small vessels in the skin or mucous membranes. They are probably not a true neoplasm, but are either congenital or an exaggeration of existing vessels.

Naevus flammeus (ordinary birthmark)
Naevus flammeus is a macular lesion with vessel dilatation. Most regress, except the 'port-wine stain' naevi, which persist and are a sign of the Sturge–Weber syndrome.

Spider naevi
Spider naevi are minute, often pulsatile arterioles occurring around a central core, usually above the waist. They are associated with hyperoestrogen states (e.g. cirrhosis and pregnancy).

Rendu–Osler–Weber disease (hereditary haemorrhagic telangiectasia)
Rendu–Osler–Weber disease is a rare autosomal dominant condition, characterized by multiple, small aneurysms on the skin and mucous membranes. Patients present with bleeding from the nose, mouth or rectum, or in urine.

Bacillary angiomatosis
Bacillary angiomatosis is a fatal disease caused by rickettsia-like bacteria. There is proliferation of blood vessels in the skin, lymph nodes, and organs of immunocompromised patients. Treatment with erythromycin is curative.

Intermediate-grade tumours
Haemangioendothelioma
Haemangioendotheliomas are neoplasms that show both benign and malignant characteristics (i.e. some are benign, others are malignant). They consist of vascular channels with masses of spindle-shaped plump cells of endothelial origin.

Malignant tumours
Angiosarcoma (haemangiosarcoma)
Angiosarcomas are rare, but very aggressive tumours that metastasize widely. They are found in skin, breast, liver, and spleen, especially in the elderly. There are small, discrete, red nodules that change into large, white masses, in which cells of all differentiations are found.

Haemangiopericytoma
Haemangiopericytoma is a malignant tumour of pericytes occurring in the lower extremities or in the retroperitoneum. About half of all these tumours metastasize.

Kaposi's sarcoma
Kaposi's sarcoma is a malignant tumour of unknown origin, but probably from lymphatic endothelium. Purple papules/plaques are found in the skin, mucosa, or viscera. Microscopically, it is composed of sheets of spindle-shaped plump cells with intermingled red blood cells and vascular channels.

There are four types of this disease, described below.

Classic Kaposi's sarcoma
Classic Kaposi's sarcoma affects mainly elderly Eastern European men, especially Ashkenazi Jews. Multiple red plaques occur on the lower extremities. The disease is rarely fatal.

African Kaposi's sarcoma
African Kaposi's sarcoma affects mainly younger men in equatorial Africa. Clinically, it is similar to classic Kaposi's sarcoma.

Transplant-associated Kaposi's sarcoma
Transplant-associated Kaposi's sarcoma occurs in immunosuppressed patients. It involves the skin and viscera. Lesions regress when immunosuppression is stopped.

HIV-associated Kaposi's sarcoma

HIV-associated Kaposi's sarcoma may occur in the skin, mucous membranes, lymph nodes, viscera, or gastrointestinal tract. This is an AIDS-defining illness, and it often responds to cytotoxic drugs or α-interferon.

Diseases of the veins and lymphatics

Varicose veins

Varicose veins are tortuous, distended superficial veins, usually of the lower limbs, caused by a persistent increased intraluminal pressure. They occur in 10–20% of the normal population, with women being more affected than men. Risk factors include:

- Pregnancy.
- Obesity.
- Prolonged standing.

- Previous deep vein thrombosis.
- Familial tendency.
- Tumours compressing the deep veins.

Aetiology

There are superficial and deep veins in the lower limb, which are interconnected by perforating veins (Fig. 5.33). Blood is returned mainly through the deep veins to the thoracic compartment by the skeletal pumping effect of the calf muscles. If there is a blockage of the deep veins (e.g. by thrombosis) or there are faulty valves in the perforating veins, then blood will move from the deep veins into the superficial veins. This will lead to distension and further valvular incompetence, resulting in stasis of blood. Oedema and changes in the skin take place (e.g. ulceration, which fails to heal because there is an impaired circulation).

Histologically, the venous walls will become thin where there is dilatation. Thrombosis may be seen in the superficial vein walls, but this rarely causes emboli.

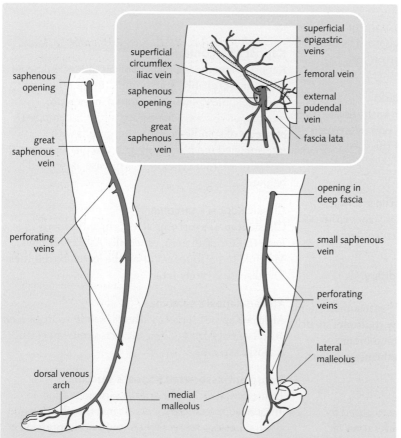

Fig. 5.33 Perforating veins of the lower limbs.

Sequelae

Sequelae of varicose veins include:

- Varicose ulcers.
- Dermatitis.
- Thromboemboli.

Other parts of the body where varicosities may occur

These are as follows:

- Haemorrhoids (piles) are distended submucosal veins in the anal canal that may protrude through the anus. Bleeding and pain may result from trauma, protrusion, or spasm of the anal sphincter.
- Varicocoele is a distension of the veins of the pampiniform plexus in the spermatic cord.
- Oesophageal varices are distended veins at the oesophageal–gastric junction. They are caused by portal hypertension, usually as a result of liver cirrhosis.

Phlebothrombosis and thrombophlebitis

Thrombosis within a vein is termed phlebothrombosis—the term 'deep vein thrombosis' is more specific. Phlebothrombosis usually causes inflammation in the wall of the vein, which is then termed thrombophlebitis. Risk factors for thrombosis include:

- Pregnancy.
- Prolonged immobilization.
- Surgery (i.e. leading to immobilization).
- Tumour.
- Local infection.
- Congestive heart failure.
- Dehydration.

Thrombosis mainly affects the following:

- Deep leg veins (90% of thromboses; 60% of hospitalized patients on autopsy). Commonly they throw off emboli that impact in the pulmonary circulation.
- Periprostatic plexus in men.
- Ovarian and pelvic veins in women.

Clinical features of thrombosis vary:

- It may be asymptomatic.
- It may present with pulmonary emboli.
- It may cause calf pain, with swelling, redness, and distended superficial veins. The affected calf is warmer, and there may be ankle oedema.
- If severe, occlusion may lead to cyanosis of the limb, severe oedema, and gangrene.

Investigation is with Doppler ultrasonography or venography. Treatment is by anticoagulation therapy with heparin. The patient is mobilized and advised to wear support stockings.

In late pregnancy, phlegmasia alba dolens (painful white 'milk leg') may occur because of thrombosis of the iliofemoral veins.

Thrombophlebitis migrans (Trousseau's syndrome) refers to multiple thrombi occurring in one place and then vanishing only to occur somewhere else. It is caused by hypercoagulability states associated with cancer.

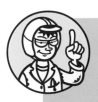

Deep vein thrombosis is often asymptomatic, but it may lead to fatal complications. Any immobile patient should be considered at risk. Long haul flights are a risk factor, even for young adults—fluid intake, aspirin and regular leg exercise will minimize risk.

Lymphangitis and lymphoedema

Lymphangitis is inflammation of the lymphatic vessels. It is frequently found in lymphatic vessels that drain a source of infection. It often presents as a cluster of red painful streaks in the skin close to an infected site. Lymphangitis very often occurs as a result of bacterial infections (especially streptococcal). If untreated with antibiotics, it may progress to involve the lymph nodes (lymphadenitis), and it may eventually lead to septicaemia.

Histologically, the wall of the lymph vessels is infiltrated by inflammatory cells. This may spread to involve surrounding structures leading to cellulitis or an abscess.

Lymphoedema is an accumulation of interstitial fluid caused by obstruction of the draining lymphatics. The oedema may be pitting initially. This may be caused by:

- Recurrent cellulitis.
- Malignancy.
- Surgical resection of lymph nodes.
- Radiotherapy causing fibrosis.
- Filariasis—nematode worm infection that leads to elephantiasis (gross enlargement of the skin and connective tissue).

113

- Post-inflammatory thrombosis leading to scarring.
- Congenital abnormal lymphatics.

If lymphoedema is prolonged, fibrosis of the interstitium occurs, leading to skin thickening and permanent oedema. The skin appears to take on an orange-peel appearance (peau d'orange). Associated ulcers and brawny hardening of the skin may also take place.

If the dilated obstructed lymphatics rupture, then chyle (lymph with digested fats) may accumulate in parts of the body cavity. Chylous ascites, chylothorax, and chylopericardium refer to the accumulation of chyle in the abdomen, thorax, and pericardium, respectively.

Neoplasms of the lymphatics
Lymphangioma
Lymphangiomas are benign tumours of the lymphatic capillaries. They are analogous to haemangiomas. There are two types: simple and cavernous.

Simple lymphangioma
Typically, a simple lymphangioma occurs on the head, neck, or axilla. It can also occur on the trunk and in viscera.

Simple lymphangiomas are cutaneous or pedunculated nodules made up of endothelium-lined spaces in a network. No blood cells are present.

Cavernous lymphangioma (cystic hygroma)
Cavernous masses are usually present in the neck or axilla in children. They are not encapsulated, and they are poorly defined so difficult to resect. Cavernous lymphangiomas tend to recur. There are dilated cystic spaces lined by endothelium.

Lymphangiosarcoma
Lymphangiosarcoma is a rare malignant tumour of the lymphatics with a poor prognosis. Prolonged lymphoedema is usually associated with the condition.

The tumour comprises multiple confluent nodules of vascular channels lined with endothelium.

Therapeutic interventions in cardiovascular disease

Direct, non-drug interventions are to be considered when:
- There is a lesion that can be treated by an appropriate technique.

- General measures and medical treatment have failed to relieve the symptoms.
- The benefits from surgery outweigh the risk of the procedure.

Treatment for arrhythmia
DC shock (cardioversion therapy)
Cardioversion therapy is used to treat serious ventricular tachycardia and fibrillation. A defibrillator is used to give a shock to the heart through the skin. This should abolish the arrhythmia and allow the sinoatrial node to take back control of the heart's rhythm. Implantable cardioverter–defibrillators (ICDs) are available that can be implanted into the body. These ICD devices detect any arrhythmia that may occur, and they give a small shock to return the rhythm to sinus rhythm. Triggered DC shock is the treatment of choice for broad QRS complex tachycardias. The shock must be delivered on the S wave of the electrocardiogram.

Pacemaker
This is often used in sick sinus syndrome where there is disease of the sinus node (ischaemia, infarction, or degeneration), leading to pauses in sinus node function or bradycardia. Pacemakers can be implanted into the body to control the heart rate. An electrode is placed in the right atrium and linked to a voltage generator. This artificial pacemaker is then set at a certain frequency such that it takes over the role of the sinoatrial node in generating cardiac depolarization.

If the atrium is fibrillating when there is heart block, a ventricular electrode is used. Heart block with intact atrial function requires a dual chamber pacemaker.

Treatment for angina
Balloon angioplasty
Balloon angioplasty (percutaneous transluminal coronary angioplasty—PTCA) uses information gained from a coronary angiogram, which shows the state of the coronary vasculature. It is usually used for the treatment of isolated, proximal, non-calcified atheromatous plaques, but it can be used for multiple lesions and it can be repeated.

The method involves the use of a balloon that is inflated in the stenosed artery to cause dilation. The balloon is inserted through the obstruction in the artery using X-ray fluoroscopy and then inflated with a contrast material. Multiple inflations of the balloon compress and crack the atheroma. This should reduce the obstruction.

Complications are:

- Acute coronary occlusion.
- Re-stenosis (occurs in 30% in first 6 months).

Outcome can be improved using a device called a stent—a metallic 'scaffold'—that is introduced around the balloon catheter. Inflation of the balloon fixes the stent in position, reducing the risk of re-stenosis.

Coronary artery bypass graft (CABG)

For left anterior descending (LAD) artery lesions, the left internal mammary artery is detached distally and anastomosed distal to the coronary artery stenosis. A vein is taken (usually from the leg), and this is used to bypass obstructions to other main coronary vessels. It is usually attached from the aorta to the artery distal to the obstruction. Multiple obstructions can by dealt with by these methods. Considerable improvement is achieved from the surgery in about 90% of cases (Fig. 5.34).

Complications are:

- Mortality (about 1%).
- Slow occlusion of the grafts.

Treatment for heart failure—heart transplantation

Heart transplantation has become the treatment of choice for severe, intractable heart failure in younger patients. Life expectancy would be about 6 months without radical intervention. The procedure requires the use of ciclosporin for immunosuppression. With good patient selection, the prognosis is good, with one-year survival rates of 80% and five-year survival of 70%. The quality of life of the majority of patients is dramatically improved.

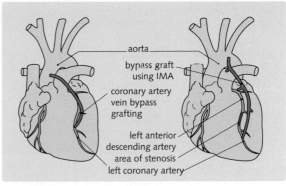

aorta
bypass graft using IMA
coronary artery vein bypass grafting
left anterior descending artery
area of stenosis
left coronary artery

Fig. 5.34 Coronary artery bypass graft using a leg vein and left internal mammary artery (IMA). (Redrawn with permission from Thelan IA, et al. *Critical Care Nursing: Diagnosis and Management*, 2nd edn. Mosby Year Book, 1994.)

Interventional procedures are generally more hazardous than non-intervention, but sometimes they can confer tremendous improvement in the patient, so that any increased risk is worth taking. For example, CABG has inherent risks in the operative procedure, but after successful completion the risk of infarction is lowered compared to that with standard medical therapy.

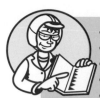

- Define shock and its causes.
- What is the clinical picture of shock?
- Describe the cardiovascular responses to haemorrhage.
- What are the causes and risk factors of hypertension?
- What are the differences between benign and malignant hypertension?
- What factors can cause pulmonary hypertension?
- List the drugs that may be used to treat hypertension. What combinations should be avoided and why?
- Describe how lipids are transported and metabolized.
- What are the main hyperlipidaemias?
- What options are available to treat hyperlipidaemias?
- What is the difference between arteriosclerosis and atherosclerosis?
- What are the risk factors of atherosclerosis, and how can these risks be reduced?
- Outline the series of pathogenic changes thought to lead to atheroma. What cells and signals are involved?
- Describe the complications of atherosclerosis.
- Why is diabetes a risk factor for atherosclerosis? What other vascular changes are associated with diabetes?
- What are the main causes and types of aneurysms?
- How would you differentiate between true and false aneurysms?
- What is aortic dissection? What are possible complications?
- What are the features of an abdominal aortic aneurysm?
- What are the syndromes of ischaemic heart disease?
- What are the risk factors and aetiology of ischaemic heart disease?
- What is the definition of angina and how is it classified?
- What is the physiological basis for the treatment of angina? List the drugs available for treatment.
- How are myocardial infarctions classified? What pathogenic changes lead to the different types?
- What treatments are available for myocardial infarction, and how do they work?
- How can sudden cardiac death result from ischaemic heart disease?
- How does cardiac failure arise? How does it present?
- How does the body attempt to compensate for cardiac failure? Are these changes helpful?
- What is the basis for the drug treatment of heart failure? How do the different drugs contribute?
- What forms of arrhythmias are there?
- What mechanisms are involved in causing arrhythmias?
- How can anti-arrhythmic drugs be classified? What are the three general aims for drug treatment, and what mechanisms are involved in achieving these effects?
- What valvular diseases are there? What are their sequelae?
- What are the causes and complications of infective endocarditis?
- Describe the pathogenesis and features of the following diseases:
  - Dilated cardiomyopathy.
  - Hypertrophic cardiomyopathy.
  - Restrictive cardiomyopathy.
  - Myocarditis.
- What is a pericardial effusion? What are its causes?
- What can cause cardiac tamponade? What can result from this?

- Describe the features of pericarditis.
- Describe the various classifications of the vasculitides.
- What are the features of giant-cell arteritis and polyarteritis nodosa?
- Describe how the following conditions arise, and how they present:
  - Atrial septal defect.
  - Ventricular septal defect.
  - Patent ductus arteriosus.
  - Fallot's tetralogy.
  - Transposition of the great arteries.
  - Coarctation of the aorta.
- What are the two important developmental anomalies of the vessels?
- What are the effects of neoplastic disease on the cardiovascular system?
- How might a primary cardiac myxoma present?
- What types of haemangioma are there?
- What are telangiectasias? What different types are there?
- Describe the features of Kaposi's sarcoma in a patient with AIDS.
- What are the risk factors for varicose veins? How do they develop, and what possible sequelae are there?
- How do deep vein thromboses occur? How can they be prevented?
- What are lymphoedema and lymphangitis? How do they arise?
- What non-drug treatments are available for arrhythmia?
- What are the uses, risks, and prognosis of angioplasty and bypass grafting?

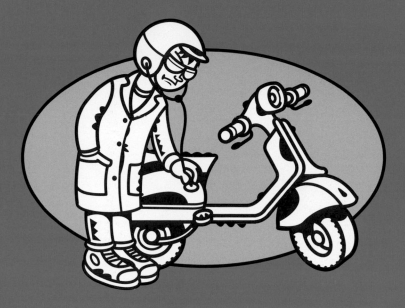

CLINICAL ASSESSMENT

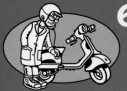

6. Common Presentations of Cardiovascular Disease

Common presenting complaints

Cardiovascular disease may present in a number of ways. Chest pain is the most obvious example, but shortness of breath or reduced exercise tolerance may be the first thing noticed by a patient. It should not be forgotten that some cardiovascular conditions may be asymptomatic, and these are diagnosed fortuitously when the patient is being examined for another complaint.

In this chapter we will discuss the common presentations of cardiovascular disease, and the differential diagnoses that they suggest.

Chest pain

When a patient presents with chest pain (Figs 6.1 and 6.2), the following points must be investigated:

- Exact site, nature and severity of pain.
- Onset.
- Duration.
- Radiation (e.g. to the arms).
- Precipitating factors (e.g. exercise).

Causes of central and lateral chest pain	
Central pain	**Lateral pain**
Cardiac Angina Myocardial infarction Pericarditis Mitral valve prolapse	Respiratory Pneumonia Pneumothorax Neoplasia Tuberculosis Connective tissue disorders
Aortic Dissecting aortic aneurysm Aortitis	Chest wall disorders (cause pleuritic pain) Rib fracture Intercostal muscle injury
Pulmonary/mediastinal Embolus Tracheitis Neoplasia	Psychogenic Anxiety
Oesophageal Oesophagitis (indigestion) Mallory–Weiss syndrome	Other Pulmonary embolus *Herpes zoster*
Traumatic	
Psychogenic	

Fig. 6.1 Causes of central and peripheral chest pain.

- Relieving factors (e.g. rest).
- Associated features.

Angina

Angina is characterized by a constricting, tightening, or choking pain on exertion that is relieved by rest or glyceryl trinitrate (GTN). The pain may radiate to the left arm and neck, and it may be exacerbated by emotion, large meals, or a cold wind.

Acute coronary syndromes

Acute coronary syndromes include unstable angina or myocardial infarction. They are characterized by a spontaneous onset of continuous intense constricting or tightening pain at rest, which may be accompanied by sweating and vomiting. The patient may be very anxious and feel that he or she is about to die (sense of impending doom).

Acute pericarditis

Acute pericarditis is characteristically described as a sharp pain, usually localized to the left of the sternum. It varies in intensity with movement and respiration.

Dissecting aortic aneurysm

A patient with a dissecting aortic aneurysm may present with severe, sharp, tearing pain radiating to the back. The pulse may be slow and asymmetrical.

Oesophageal pain

Oesophageal pain often mimics angina—it may be precipitated by exercise, and it may be relieved with GTN. It may be described as a burning pain with a history related to food intake or oesophageal reflux.

Aortic stenosis and hypertrophic obstructive cardiomyopathy

These two conditions may also mimic angina.

Dyspnoea (shortness of breath)

How short of breath is the patient? Is the dyspnoea brought on by exercise or is the patient short of breath at rest? How much exercise brings it on (ask about dressing, climbing stairs, and walking). Dyspnoea may be caused by:

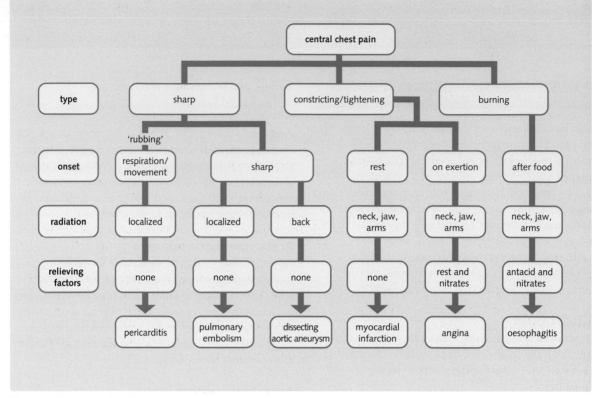

Fig. 6.2 Chest pain algorithm.

The algorithms for presenting complaints are only a general guide to establishing a diagnosis. Many complaints may strongly indicate a particular diagnosis, but the patient might have a different problem—for example the patient may present with a burning central chest pain after eating; this may be indigestion, but it might be a mild myocardial infarction. Remember that medicine is not an exact science; you are always dealing in probability. The diagnosis will need to be confirmed with an investigation (e.g. measure levels of creatine kinase).

- Heart failure if associated with orthopnoea, paroxysmal nocturnal dyspnoea (PND), or oedema.

- Mitral stenosis.
- Shock.
- Respiratory causes (e.g. asthma, pulmonary embolism, pneumothorax).

Orthopnoea

Orthopnoea is shortness of breath while lying flat. It indicates left heart failure. Ask the patient 'Can you lie flat to sleep?' 'Do you need to prop yourself up with pillows?' 'How many?'

Paroxysmal nocturnal dyspnoea

Paroxysmal nocturnal dyspnoea (PND) is a sudden shortness of breath at night, causing the patient to awaken. It indicates left heart failure. Ask the patient 'Do you get attacks of breathlessness that wake you up at night?' 'How do you get over it?'

Oedema

Ask the patient 'Have you noticed any swelling in your feet or ankles?' Peripheral oedema is an indication of:
- Congestive cardiac failure—oedema indicates the characteristic fluid retention of heart failure.
- Venous thrombosis.

- Lymphoedema (caused by Milroy's syndrome, radiotherapy, malignancy, or infection) if the oedema is non-pitting (i.e. when you press the skin, no indentation remains).
- Other diseases (e.g. liver disease, nephrotic syndrome etc.).

Hypertension

The World Health Organization definition of hypertension is blood pressure higher than 140 mmHg systolic or 90 mmHg diastolic in the elderly (see p.74). Blood pressure must be elevated on more than one examination for the patient to be diagnosed as hypertensive. If no organ damage is indicated, then blood pressure measurements should be taken over a long period of time before a diagnosis of hypertension is reached. Mild hypertension is usually asymptomatic.

Secondary causes of hypertension are suggested by a specific history (e.g. sweating and tachycardia suggest phaeochromocytoma).

Malignant hypertension often presents with:
- Visual impairment.
- Nausea and vomiting.
- Fits.
- Transient paralysis.
- Severe headaches.
- Impairment of consciousness.
- Symptoms of cardiac failure.
- Angina (due to atherosclerosis or high oxygen demand from hypertrophied myocardium).

Hypotension

Hypotension results if the systolic blood pressure falls below 80 mmHg. It often presents with the classic features of shock (tachycardia and cold, clammy skin, etc.). Hypotension can be caused by:
- Anaphylactic, cardiogenic, or septicaemic shock.
- Volume depletion (hypovolaemic shock)—haemorrhage, burns, gastrointestinal losses (vomiting or diarrhoea), renal losses (diuretic therapy, nephropathy, diabetes mellitus).
- Drugs and drug overdose—opiates, barbiturates, amphetamines, antidepressants.

Commonly, postural hypotension results. This is a fall in blood pressure on standing (blood pressure should normally rise because of venoconstriction in the legs). The causes of postural hypotension are:
- Volume depletion.
- Autonomic failure (caused by diabetes mellitus or amyloidosis).

- Drugs that interfere with autonomic function (e.g. ganglion blockers or tricyclic antidepressants).
- Interference with peripheral venoconstriction by drugs (e.g. nitrates, calcium antagonists, α-blockers).
- Prolonged bed rest.

Heart murmurs

If a patient with heart murmurs is cyanosed, a shunt may be present. Ask whether the patient can feel a thrill (a murmur you can palpate with your hand). Note whether the murmur is causing the patient any distress.

Listen to the murmur in the auscultatory areas and decide where the murmur is in relation to the cardiac cycle. Listen for intensity, any radiation, and any other associated sounds. Diastolic murmurs should be considered to be a serious sign. For more details and a differential diagnosis see Chapter 7.

Syncope (fainting)

Ask the patient whether they have ever fainted. The following points should be noted.
- Onset.
- Any loss of consciousness.
- Any warning (aura).
- Light-headedness or vertigo beforehand.
- Duration.
- Any memory loss.
- Any injuries sustained during the faint.
- Any incontinence.

Syncope can be caused by:
- Vasovagal attack—a powerful centrally mediated reflex, initiated by pain, powerful emotional stimulus, or sudden underperfusion of the brain (see Chapter 4).
- Stokes–Adams attack—a transient arrhythmia that causes a loss of cardiac output. Usually, there is no warning (but possible palpitations). Causes pallor, and an irregular or slow pulse.
- Aortic stenosis or intracardiac thrombus/tumour—produces a similar picture.
- Postural hypotension—occurs when suddenly standing.
- Carotid sinus syndrome—occurs in patients aged over 50 years while turning their head. Can be checked for by massaging one of the carotids while feeling for extreme bradycardia.
- Vertebrobasilar insufficiency—also occurs while turning the head.

- Respiratory causes—cough syncope or anxiety with hyperventilation.
- Other causes—hypoglycaemia, raised intracranial pressure, or alcohol/drug ingestion.

Do not forget to exclude epilepsy.

Abnormalities of heart rate and rhythm
Palpitations
Note any instances of palpitations. Ask 'Do you ever notice your heart beat?' 'Does it go really fast?' 'Can you tap it out on the table for me?' Palpitations are caused by:

- Arrhythmias. A regularly irregular pulse indicates intermittent heart block or ectopic beats, an irregularly irregular pulse indicates atrial fibrillation.
- Anxiety.

Intermittent claudication
Intermittent claudication is an indication of peripheral vascular disease impeding arterial flow in the legs. You should ask the patient 'Do you get cramp-like pain in your legs while walking or at rest?' 'How far can you walk?' 'How long do you have to rest to allow the pain to go away?' 'Can you walk the same distance after you've stopped?'

Elevated serum cholesterol and triglycerides
Hyperlipidaemic patients might present with the following conditions or signs:

- Xanthoma (lipid deposits in a tendon).
- Xanthelasma or corneal arcus (lipid deposits in the cornea).
- Obesity.
- Hypertension.
- Pancreatitis.
- Diabetes mellitus.

Patients may also have a family history of lipid disorders or coronary heart disease. Secondary causes of hyperlipidaemia must be excluded. These include:

- Hypothyroidism.
- Diabetes mellitus.
- Obesity.
- Renal impairment.
- Nephrotic syndrome.
- Liver dysfunction.
- Dysglobulinaemia.
- Drugs (especially oral contraceptives, thiazides, corticosteroids).

A good method to use if you are stuck for a diagnosis is to employ a surgical sieve. This is a methodical approach to obtaining differential diagnoses by considering systems. Usually the first approach is to consider congenital and acquired causes. The acquired causes are further subdivided. A mnemonic for this is 'TIN CAN BED MD':
T—trauma
I—infection
N—neoplasia
C—connective tissue disorders
A—arterial and venous disease
N—nervous system
B—blood disorders
E—endocrine
D—drugs
M—metabolic disorders
D—deficiency

- List the questions that you should ask to fully characterize a patient's report of chest pain.
- What are the presenting features of angina, myocardial infarction, heart failure, and pericarditis? How do they differ?
- What are the differential diagnoses for a patient presenting with chest pain?
- What can cause dyspnoea?
- What can cause oedema?
- How would a patient present with severe malignant hypertension?
- How would a patient present with hypotension? What would cause this condition?
- What can cause syncope?
- What other symptoms may indicate cardiovascular disease?
- What signs or symptoms may indicate a hyperlipidaemia?

7. History and Examination

Taking a history

Important points to remember when taking a history include observation, introduction, and communication. These are discussed in more detail below.

Observation

Have a look around the bed for clues as to the patient's condition. (Are there inhalers on the bedside table? Are there walking aids in the room? Are there intravenous drips, oxygen bottles, or monitors?)

Make an initial assessment of the patient. (Is the patient in distress, finding it hard to breathe? How many pillows is the patient using?)

This assessment should continue and be updated throughout the interview.

Introduction

Always greet the patient and introduce yourself, explaining who you are and what you are about to do. Try to shake the patient's hand. This is not only normal politeness, but it also allows you to ascertain some of the motor functions of their hand.

Ensure that the patient is comfortable at all times. Be prepared to halt the interview if circumstances warrant (e.g. the patient might want to go to the toilet, or lunch might arrive). Remember you can always come back later.

If there are relatives around, do not be afraid to ask them to leave to allow you to talk privately. Obviously, if the relative has only just got there or has only got a limited time with the patient, then you must come back at a more appropriate time. Most of the time, however, relatives are happy for you to interrupt them because it is an excuse for them to have a break.

If there are other people with the patient while you are taking a history (this can be daunting initially), you can use them to corroborate or give a different view on the information presented. Sensitive questions can be reserved until the examination when you will be alone with the patient.

Communication
Non-verbal communication

Sit down at a comfortable distance from the patient. Give the patient your full attention and make only brief notes.

Listen to what the patient is saying rather than just writing it down; you will then pick up on comments that can lead to further questions. This is harder than it sounds as frequently you are concentrating so hard on trying to think of the next question that you do not hear a vital clue. Keep the conversation flowing by nodding at appropriate moments.

Verbal communication

Ask open-ended questions ('What was the pain like?') rather than leading ones ('Was it a crushing pain?').

Let patients answer questions in their own words, without interruption. You should be aiming to hold a conversation rather than performing an interrogation. If you feel that the patient is rambling, gently try to steer the conversation back with a direct question ('If I could just clarify what the pain was like . . . ?').

Try not to use medical terms (e.g. for orthopnoea, ask 'How many pillows do you need to get to sleep?').

If a patient says he has a certain condition, ask him to explain what he understands it to be and how it affects him. Beware of terms like 'gastric flu'. What does the patient mean by this?

Use phrases like 'yes', 'a-ha', and 'I see' to help the conversation flow.

Overall, try to be friendly and confident and attempt to make the patient feel at ease. Do not be too worried if you cannot reach a diagnosis, but try to think of what the problem could be.

Presenting complaint

The presenting complaint is a symptom felt by the patient and not a diagnosis.

There may be more than one complaint, in which case, number the symptoms and take a history for each complaint.

History of the presenting complaint

Generally you need to find out the following information:
- Nature of the complaint.
- Site of the complaint.
- Extent of the deficit. How disabling is it?
- Onset. What time during the day? Which activities bring it on?
- Course. How does the symptom pattern vary? What is the frequency—is it intermittent or continuous?
- Duration. How long has it been there?
- Precipitating and relieving factors.
- Other relevant symptoms.
- Any previous treatment or investigations for this same complaint.

You should usually let the patient tell you the natural history of the complaint, but symptoms you should specifically ask about are:
- Chest pain.
- Shortness of breath, orthopnoea, and paroxysmal nocturnal dyspnoea (PND).
- Oedema.
- Palpitations.
- Syncope (fainting) or dizziness.
- Intermittent claudication.
- Other symptoms—any coldness, redness, or blueness of the extremities (symptoms of peripheral vascular disease); sweating; fever; appetite change, nausea, or vomiting (symptoms of heart failure or digitalis toxicity); tiredness (might be caused by heart failure or ischaemia, or may be a consequence of treatment such as β-blockers).
- Smoking.

Past medical history

Ask the patient if they have any other medical problems. Then say 'I'm going to run through a list of conditions to make sure we don't miss anything out – you might say "No" to most of these . . .'.

Important past medical conditions to note include:
- Diabetes mellitus.
- Hypertension.
- Myocardial infarction.
- Stroke (cerebrovascular accident—CVA).
- Angina.
- Arrhythmia.
- Peripheral vascular disease.
- Rheumatic fever.

- Intermittent claudication.
- Renal failure.

Previous operations to note include:
- Coronary artery bypass graft (CABG).
- Angioplasty.
- Pacemaker insertion.
- Vascular surgery.

Drug history

A note should be made of all prescription and over-the-counter medications that are currently being used. Aspects of the presenting complaint may be due to current therapy. Be aware that some herbal and alternative medications have pharmacological effects or interactions (e.g. St John's wort and digoxin).

Any allergies should be noted, especially those due to drugs. To establish whether a true anaphylactic reaction takes place, ask the patient what happens when they come into contact with the substance.

Family history

Any relevant family history should be noted. Ask whether there is any incidence of the following diseases in close relatives:
- Diabetes mellitus.
- Myocardial infarction.
- CVA.
- Angina.
- Hypertension.
- Any hereditary disorder.

Find out the state of health of the patient's father, mother, siblings, and children. If they have died, ask what they died of and at what age, but remember to be sensitive.

Social history

Enquire into the patient's marital status and children. Note the patient's present living conditions and any problems that these may cause (e.g. 'are there many steps that the patient cannot negotiate?'). Life-style, including diet and exercise, should be elicited:
- If the patient smokes, find out how many per day, and for how many years.
- How much alcohol is taken? How often? It is notoriously difficult to get an accurate history of alcohol consumption: often, you must ask questions like 'How long does a bottle of whisky last you?'.
- Has the patient ever taken any illicit drugs?
- Ask if the patient has travelled abroad recently.

You might also need to ask about sexual practices.

Occupational history

A careful occupational history should not be neglected. Find out the patient's current and previous employment, with particular emphasis on levels of stress and industrial exposure to chemicals or physical agents. Be aware that patients may be worried about the consequences of their health on their job, and that there are medicolegal implications with certain careers (e.g. commercial driver, pilot).

 If a patient mentions an unfamiliar procedure or treatment, don't be afraid to ask the patient why they think they received that treatment. This will also help you to give better explanations in future.

Review of systems

This is a systematic review of the whole body in an attempt to elicit any other symptoms. Points to note are outlined below.

Respiratory system

Note the presence of any cough or sputum. This may indicate pulmonary oedema, and it is also a side effect of angiotensin-converting enzyme (ACE) inhibitors.

Gastrointestinal system

Epigastric pain might be caused by a myocardial infarction. Other abdominal pain might be caused by an aortic aneurysm (if it ruptures, there may be continuous abdominal pain) or ischaemia of the mesenteric vessels.

Increased thirst, if associated with other signs, may indicate dehydration, possibly caused by haemorrhage or shock.

Genitourinary system

Causes of increased frequency of micturition and increased urine production include diabetes mellitus and diuretic therapy. Intermittent tachycardias may also cause increased urine production. Nocturia (needing to micturate at night) may be caused by heart failure.

Musculoskeletal system

Joint pain can indicate a systemic disorder with cardiac effects (e.g. systemic lupus erythematosus).

Nervous system

A note should be made of:
- Any visual disturbances (e.g amaurosis fugax— 'seeing curtains drawn across the eye').
- Temporary blindness (due to emboli reaching the retinal vessels and causing ischaemia of the retina—these emboli can arise from atheromatous plaques).

Observation of the whole body

General appearance

Note the general appearance of the patient. Is the patient:
- Well/ill/distressed?
- Alert/confused?
- Happy/sad?
- Thin/fat?

Colour

Look at the skin. Note any evidence of:
- Pallor/anaemia—pale skin.
- Cyanosis/shock—blueish tinge.

These may imply:
- Hypovolaemia to skin.
- Peripheral vascular disease.
- Pulmonary to systemic shunting.
- Lung disease.
- Haemoglobinopathy.

Rash

Look at any rash. Note size, type—macula (flat) or papula (raised), colour, surface, and reaction to pressure—does it blanch or not?

Gross abnormalities
Marfan syndrome

Marfan syndrome is usually an autosomal dominant inherited condition. Those with the syndrome show the following signs:
- Elongated and asymmetrical face.
- Dislocation of the lens of the eye (ectopia lentis).
- High-arched palate.

- Tall, with lower half of body larger than the upper half. The arm span is usually longer than the height.
- Long thin digits (arachnodactyly).

Degeneration of vessel media can lead to a dissecting aneurysm in the ascending aorta, which may rupture. An incompetent mitral valve may also result.

Down syndrome

Down syndrome is trisomy of chromosome 21. Those with the syndrome show the following signs:
- Flat face with slanting eyes and epicanthic folds.
- Small ears.
- Simian crease (single plantar crease on the palm).
- Short, stubby fingers.
- Hypotonia.

There is a variable level of mental retardation. Up to 50% of children with Down syndrome have a congenital heart defect; the most common is an atrioventricular septal defect, followed by a ventricular septal defect.

Turner's syndrome

In Turner's syndrome, the genotype is XO (female). Those with the syndrome show infantilism (appear childlike even when an adult), a webbed neck, short stature, cubitus valgus (increased carrying angle of elbow), and primary amenorrhoea (no menstrual bleeding).

Intelligence is normal. Other features can include coarctation of the aorta and other left-sided heart defects and lymphoedema of the legs.

In an examination, if you are making a general inspection, make it obvious to the examiner.

The limbs

Fig. 7.1 gives details of hand examination.

There are few signs to note in the arms and forearms. However, the radial and brachial pulses must be assessed (see below).

Fig. 7.2 gives details of examination of the lower limb.

Adopt a system for doing the examination. For example, always examine in the following order:
- Inspection, then palpation, percussion, and auscultation of each area that you are examining.
- Examine the hands, then the upper limbs, neck, face, chest, and abdomen; then, examine the lower limbs.

Ensure that you use the same method when examining every patient with cardiovascular symptoms. In this way, you will not miss any signs.

Peripheral arterial pulses

Pulses should be checked as a matter of routine on all patients. Pulses on both sides of the body should be checked and compared. Blood pressure should be measured as outlined in Chapter 3.

Radial pulse

Palpate the radial pulse with the tips of the fingers and gently compress the radial artery against the head of the radius. This pulse is often used to assess heart rate and rhythm. The pulse character is best assessed at the carotid. After locating the pulse, wait a while before counting the rate. The rate should be counted for about 30 s and then doubled to give a rate per minute. A normal pulse is between 60–100 beats per minute (bpm). Outside this range is bradycardia (<60 bpm) or tachycardia (>100 bpm). The rhythm may be regular or irregular; if it is irregular, note whether it is a repeating irregularity (regularly irregular) or is completely irregular (irregularly irregular):
- Regular. Normal rhythm—remember sinus arrhythmia is normal (an increased rate during inspiration).
- Regularly irregular. Commonly caused by ectopic systolic beats or second-degree heart block (see Chapters 5 and 8).
- Irregularly irregular. Usually caused by atrial fibrillation or multiple ectopic beats (see Chapter 5).

Examination of the hands			
Area	Sign observed	Test performed	Diagnostic inference
Nails	Clubbing (loss of the angle at the base of the nail) 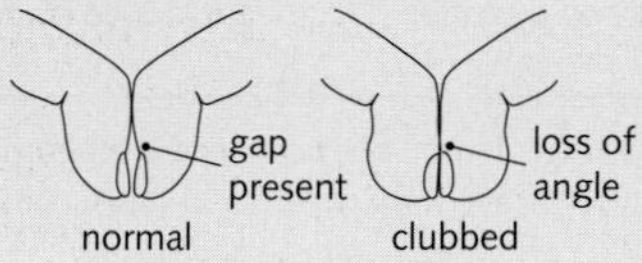 gap present — normal loss of angle — clubbed	Hold nails of both hands together and facing each other; if there is a gap, there is no clubbing	Infective endocarditis and cyanotic congenital heart disease Other causes: bronchial carcinoma, bronchial empyema/abscess, bronchiectasis, cystic fibrosis, fibrosing alveolitis, mesothelioma, Crohn's disease, cirrhosis, coeliac disease, gastrointestinal lymphoma
	Splinter haemorrhages (small, linear, haemorrhages under the nail that are splinter-like) 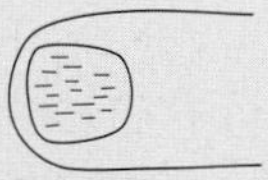	—	Infective endocarditis; commonly found after trauma to the nail, especially in manual workers
Fingers	Nicotine stains	—	Smoking
	Osler's nodes (red, painful, transient swellings on pulp of fingers and toes)	—	Infective endocarditis
Palms	Janeway lesions (small, erythematous macules on the thenar and hypothenar eminences that blanch under pressure)	—	Infective endocarditis
Dorsum	Palmar xanthomas (lipid-like deposits in the skin creases)	—	Type III hyperlipidaemia (increased intermediate density lipoproteins)
	Tendon xanthomas (yellow nodules over the extensor tendons)	—	Familial hypercholesterolaemia

Fig. 7.1 Examination of the hands. Finger clubbing is an important sign of disease, and it should always be checked for. Clubbing is demonstrated by abnormal curvature of the nail, fluctuation of the nail bed and loss of the angle between the nail bed and the nail itself.

The volume of the pulse should be assessed. A low volume implies a decreased cardiac output. A high volume pulse (described as bounding) may be caused by conditions including anaemia, carbon dioxide retention, liver disease, or thyrotoxicosis.

Radioradial delay is delay of the left radial pulse compared with the right: this may be due to coarctation of the aorta proximal to the left subclavian artery.

Brachial pulse

Palpate just above the medial aspect of the antecubital fossa and compress the brachial artery against the humerus. If you have trouble, palpate the tendon of biceps and move your fingers medial to it. Use your left hand to measure the patient's right brachial pulse and the right hand to measure the left brachial pulse.

Carotid pulse

The carotid pulse should be palpated by pressing backwards at the medial border of the sternocleidomastoid and lateral to the thyroid cartilage. The left thumb should be used to palpate the patient's right carotid pulse and the right thumb used for the left pulse. The two pulses should never be palpated at the same time or you will risk restricting the cerebral blood supply. Make sure that

Examination of the limbs			
Area	**Sign observed**	**Test performed**	**Diagnostic inference**
Upper and lower limbs	Varicose veins (distended, tortuous, veins; usually affects the saphenous veins)	Assess if they are hard (thrombosed) or tender (phlebitis) by palpation	Thrombophlebitis may indicate a deep vein occlusion; prolonged standing
Ankle	Oedema	Press one finger in one place for one minute; see if the impression disappears quickly (normal) or not (pitting oedema)	Fluid retention Congestive cardiac failure Lymphoedema Deep vein occlusion Liver disease Nephrotic syndrome
Venous ulcer	Ulcers (breakdown of the skin that becomes very difficult to heal; venous: around medial malleolus; arterial: heel or toes) Xanthomas (itchy, yellow, eruptive nodules with red edge on extensor surfaces e.g. buttocks) Tendon xanthomas on extensor tendons		Deep vein occlusion Arterial disease Sickle cell anaemia Diabetes mellitus vasculitides (polyarteritis nodosum) Squamous cell carcinoma skin lesion Hypertriglyceridaemia Lipoprotein lipase deficiency Familial hypercholesterolaemia
Leg	Problem with sapheno-femoral junction valve	Trendelenburg test; lie patient down and raise leg; place two fingers 5 cm below femoral pulse (sapheno-femoral junction); get patient to stand with fingers still in place; release fingers; if veins fill quickly then valve is incompetent	Incompetent sapheno-femoral junction valve

Fig. 7.2 Examination of the limbs.

there is no hypersensitivity of the carotid sinus that may cause a reflex bradycardia.

The carotid pulse should be used to assess the character of the pulse (Fig. 7.3). This is difficult and there are also slight variations of normal. The important pulses to note are:

- Slow rising pulse. The pulse rises slowly to a peak and then falls slowly. It is of small volume. This indicates aortic stenosis.
- Collapsing (water-hammer) pulse. There is a rapid rise to the pulse and then a rapid fall. It is usually found in aortic regurgitation. It may also be found in patent ductus arteriosus, ruptured sinus of Valsalva, or large arteriovenous communications.
- Bisferiens pulse. This is a combination of a slow rising and collapsing pulse. It is indicative of aortic stenosis and regurgitation (incompetence).

- Pulsus bigeminus. Ectopic beats occur after every normal beat, but are too weak to be palpable, giving the appearance of a very slow pulse.
- Pulsus alternans. This is composed of alternating strong and weak pulses. It indicates severe left ventricular disease.
- Pulsus paradoxus. This is a pulse that is weaker or even disappears on inspiration. It can be a variation of normal. There is pulmonary venous distension caused by negative intrathoracic pressure on inspiration. This leads to a fall in stroke volume and, therefore, cardiac output. (When the heart rate increases to compensate it gives rise to sinus arrhythmia.) If severe, this may indicate asthma, cardiac tamponade, or pericarditis.

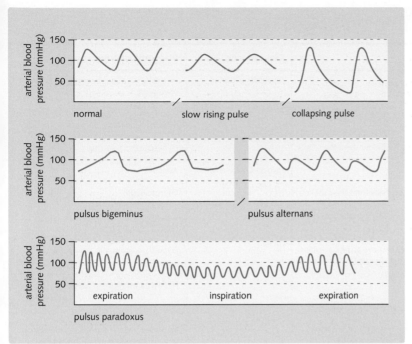

Fig. 7.3 Types of pulses. The various pulse waveforms that can result are shown here.

You should also listen in with the stethoscope diaphragm over the carotid pulse to detect any bruits (noise caused by turbulent blood flow). These may indicate that the arterial lumen has been narrowed by atheroma formation. Note, however, that the sound of turbulent flow can be heard far away from its source.

Popliteal pulse
The popliteal arteries can be found in the popliteal fossae behind the knee and are very hard to palpate. The thumbs of both hands should be rested on either side of the patella and the fingertips should be placed deep into the popliteal fossa. The popliteals are best palpated with the knees flexed at about 120 degrees.

Posterior tibial pulse
The posterior tibial pulse is palpated about 1 cm behind the medial malleolus of the tibia with the patient's foot relaxed.

Dorsalis pedis pulse
The dorsalis pedis pulse is palpated against the tarsal bones on the dorsum of the foot.

Head and neck

Face
Fig. 7.4 describes the examination of the face.

Examining the fundus of the eye is a very hard skill to master. See if you can get an ophthalmologist or senior registrar to go over what you are looking for.

Neck
Carotid pulses
The carotid pulse should be examined when taking all the other pulses.

Jugular venous pressure
The internal jugular vein will reflect the right atrial pressure. You must observe the maximum height of the jugular venous pressure (JVP) and the character of the venous pulse as follows:
1. Place the patient at a 45 degree angle, with the neck supported to relax the neck muscles. You may need to turn the patient's neck laterally.
2. Observe the junction of the sternocleidomastoid with the clavicle and then look up along the route of the jugular veins to see if you can see any visible pulsations.
3. Try palpating the pulse. If you can feel it, then the pulse is probably from the carotid artery. Venous pulses are almost impossible to feel.

	Examination of the face		
Area	**Sign observed**	**Test performed**	**Diagnostic inference**
Eyes	Jaundice	Inspect the sclerae	Hepatitis; cirrhosis; haemolysis; biliary obstruction
	Cataracts (opacities in the lens)	—	Ageing/injury; diabetes mellitus; hypercholesterolaemia
	Xanthelasma (lipid deposits above or below the eye)	—	Hypercholesterolaemia
	Pallor	Inspect conjunctivae	Anaemia
	Exophthalmos (protrusion of the eyeballs from their sockets)	—	Thyrotoxicosis
	Corneal arcus (crescenteric opacity in the periphery of the cornea)	—	Common in old people; type IV hyperlipoproteinaemia
	Lid lag (eyelid reacts much slower than eye gaze; i.e. when the patient looks up the eyelid is still drooped)	—	Hyperthyroidism
Pupils	Unequal	—	Unilateral nerve lesion; syphilis
	Irregular	—	Iritis; syphilis
	Hutchinson pupils (pupil on side of lesion constricts then widely dilates; then the other pupil does the same)	—	Increased unilateral intracranial pressure (e.g. intracerebral haemorrhage)
	Argyll–Robertson pupils (pupillary light reflex is absent but reacts to accommodation)	Pupillary light reflex	Syphilis; diabetes mellitus
Retina	Microaneurysm (small vascular leaks caused by capillary occlusion)	Fundoscopy using ophthalmoscope	Diabetes mellitus
	Hard exudates (yellow lipid deposits in the retina)		Diabetes mellitus
	Cotton-wool spots (white exudate around the macula)		Hypertension; arterial occlusion
	Flame-shaped haemorrhages (haemorrhage around optic disc spreading outwards)		Hypertension
	Retinal arteriosclerosis (copper-wire appearance of tortuous arterial vessels; nipping/indentation of veins as they cross arteries; white plaques on arteries)		Hypertension; general process associated with ageing
	Papilloedema (swelling of the optic nerve head caused by raised intracranial pressure)		Malignant hypertension; chronic meningitis; brain tumour or abscess; subdural haematoma
	Roth's spots		Infective endocarditis
Skin	Malar flush (peripheral cyanosis on cheeks)	—	Mitral stenosis
Lips	Peripheral cyanosis (bluish or purple tinge to lips)	(Unreliable sign of central cyanosis; therefore, also check the tongue)	
Tongue	Central cyanosis	—	Pulmonary–systemic shunting; lung disease; haemoglobinopathy
Palate	High-arched	—	Marfan syndrome

Fig. 7.4 Examination of the face. Generally this is restricted to just inspection unless other systems are also being assessed.

Furthermore, the venous pulse is usually complex, with a dominant inward wave, whereas the arterial pulse is usually a simple dominant outward wave. The jugular venous pressure also decreases with inspiration.

4. Estimate the vertical height of the pulse from the manubriosternal angle.

The external jugular vein is often easier to see, as it is lateral to the sternocleidomastoid and more superficial. However, it is an unreliable indicator of central venous pressure. It contains valves and moves through many fascial planes, and so it is affected by compression from structures in the neck (Fig. 7.5).

A raised jugular venous pressure is usually indicative of:

- Heart failure.
- Superior vena cava obstruction (this also abolishes any pulsations).
- Increased blood volume (e.g. pregnancy, acute nephritis, excess fluid therapy).

If the jugular venous pressure rises on inspiration (Kussmaul's sign) then consider:

- Constrictive pericarditis.
- Cardiac tamponade.

If the jugular venous pressure is normal, variation in the venous pressure waveform should be observed with the patient lying flat (Fig. 7.6).

If the jugular venous pulse is not visible, you may attempt to elicit hepatojugular reflux. This involves pushing on the liver, which should raise venous pressure and cause the jugular venous pressure to rise. You should place your hand on the right upper quadrant of the abdomen just below the ribs and push down into the abdomen and up under the

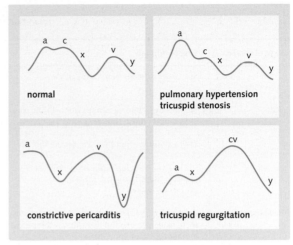

Fig. 7.6 The jugular venous pressure waveform in disease. (a, a wave—produced by atrial systole; c, c wave—caused by transmission of increasing right ventricular pressure before closure of the tricuspid valve; v, v wave—develops as right atrium fills during ventricular systole; x, x descent—occurs at end of atrial contraction; y, y descent—follows the v wave on opening of the tricuspid valve.)

ribcage, which will compress the liver against the diaphragm. The jugular venous pulse may then become visible. If the jugular venous pressure was originally so raised that it was not visible in the neck (i.e. the venous pulse was in the jaw), then this manoeuvre will not elicit any change.

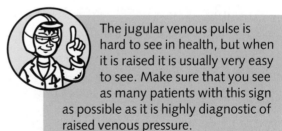

The jugular venous pulse is hard to see in health, but when it is raised it is usually very easy to see. Make sure that you see as many patients with this sign as possible as it is highly diagnostic of raised venous pressure.

Auscultation

Remember to listen over the carotid vessels—see above.

Thorax

Inspection

Fig. 7.7 describes inspection of the thorax.

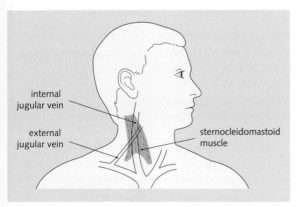

Fig. 7.5 The course of the internal and external jugular veins.

internal jugular vein

external jugular vein

sternocleidomastoid muscle

Inspection of the thorax		
Sign observed	**Test performed**	**Diagnostic inference**
Chest deformity	See *Crash Course! Respiratory System*	Bear the deformity in mind when assessing other factors (e.g. apex beat)
Scars	Sternotomy—midline scar in line with the sternum indicating that the thoracic cavity has been opened	Sternum has been cut for surgery on the heart or oesophagus
	Thoracotomy—operative scar on the thorax	Sternum has been cut for surgery on the heart or oesophagus
Masses	Lump in the left subcostal region	Pacemaker
Pulsations	Cardiac impulse; the apex beat can sometimes be seen; usually it is in the fifth intercostal space and in the midclavicular line (see Fig. 7.9)	Normal; if displaced, can indicate left ventricular hypertrophy
Rarer pulsations	Diffuse pulsation not timed with apex beat	Left ventricular aneurysm
	Pulsation to the left of sternum	Aneurysm of the descending aorta
	Suprasternal notch pulsation	Aneurysm of the arch of aorta
	Pulsation to the right of sternum	Aneurysm of the ascending aorta
	Pulsation over scapula	Coarctation of aorta

Fig. 7.7 Inspection of the thorax.

Palpation

Fig. 7.8 describes palpation of the thorax. Palpation is usually performed with the patient lying at 45 degrees. Fig. 7.9 shows the normal position of the apex beat.

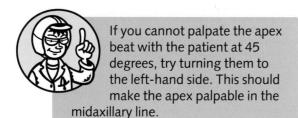

If you cannot palpate the apex beat with the patient at 45 degrees, try turning them to the left-hand side. This should make the apex palpable in the midaxillary line.

Percussion

Percussion can be useful. Percuss over the position of the heart, and define the area of cardiac dullness. A normal area of cardiac dullness does not reveal much. However, an increased area of cardiac dullness indicates cardiac enlargement or pericardial effusion. A reduced area of cardiac dullness indicates lung overinflation.

Auscultation

The stethoscope has two ends, the bell and the diaphragm (this is the larger, flatter end). The diaphragm is better for listening to higher pitched sounds; therefore, it is best for hearing:

- First and second heart sounds.
- Systolic murmurs.
- Aortic diastolic murmurs (aortic incompetence).
- Opening snap of valves.

The bell of the stethoscope is best for low-pitched sounds. The bell should not be placed too tightly to the skin, as it will then function as a diaphragm. It is used to hear:

- Third and fourth heart sounds.
- Mitral diastolic sounds (mitral stenosis).

There are certain areas where auscultation should be performed (Fig. 7.10); these are the areas where murmurs from heart valves are best heard:

- Mitral area (and axilla if murmur present).
- Tricuspid area.
- Aortic area (and neck if murmur present).

Palpation of the thorax		
Sign observed	**Test performed**	**Diagnostic inference**
Position of apex beat (Fig. 7.9)	Place hand across the chest and feel with the tips of your fingers for the lateral edge of the pulsating apex	—
—	If the apex beat is not palpable, turn the patient on to the left side and then palpate in the anterior axillary line	—
Prominent apex beat	—	Left ventricular hypertrophy
Displaced apex beat medially	—	Lung collapse; lung fibrosis
Displaced apex beat laterally apex beat more lateral	—	Left ventricular enlargement; pleural effusion; pneumothorax
Thrusting, displaced apex beat forceful and lateral, downward movement of apex	—	Volume overload: mitral/aortic incompetence
Sustained apex beat forceful and sustained impulse, which is not displaced	—	Pressure overload: aortic stenosis; hypertension; left ventricular hypertrophy
Failed detection of apex beat	—	Obesity; obstructed airways disease (overinflated); pleural effusion; pericardial effusion; dextrocardia (very rare)
Parasternal heave pulsation at left base of sternum	Palpate praecordium	Right ventricular hypertrophy
Other pulsations noted on observation (see above)	—	—
Tapping apex beat, palpable first heart sound	—	Mitral stenosis
Palpable second heart sound	—	Systemic or pulmonary hypertension
Thrills	Palpable murmurs, which feel like the purring of a cat	—
Systolic thrills in aortic area	—	Aortic stenosis
Systolic thrill at apex	—	Mitral regurgitation
Diastolic thrill	—	Mitral stenosis; aortic regurgitation (uncommon)

Fig. 7.8 Palpation of the thorax.

- Pulmonary area.
- The back.

Also use the diaphragm to auscultate the lungs from the patient's back, to check for signs of pulmonary oedema (see *Crash Course: Respiratory System*). Check for signs of lumbrosacral oedema.

Normal heart sounds

Many sounds can be heard with the stethoscope. Try to concentrate on hearing the heart sounds first (Fig. 7.11). There should be a sort of repetitive 'lupp-dubb'. Auscultating while palpating the carotid pulse will help to distinguish the heart sounds.

The first heart sound (S_1) coincides with the onset of systole and, therefore, the pulse. It is caused by the closure of the mitral and tricuspid valves. S_1 is commonly labelled M_1T_1 to reflect its two sources. The second heart sound (S_2) coincides with the beginning of diastole and it is from the closure of the aortic and pulmonary valves. The

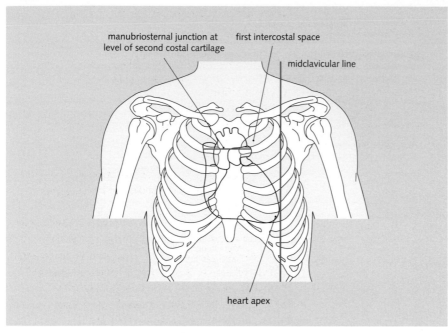

Fig. 7.9 Position of the apex beat. The apex beat is the position most inferior and furthest lateral that the cardiac impulse can be felt. As a guide to identifying intercostal spaces, the second rib lies lateral to the manubriosternal angle; the second intercostal space is below this rib. The lateral position can also be described relative to the anterior axillary line and the midaxillary line. The normal apex beat lies in the 5th intercostal space, midclavicular line.

manubriosternal junction at level of second costal cartilage

first intercostal space

midclavicular line

heart apex

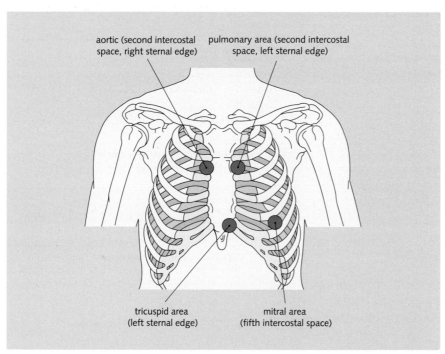

Fig. 7.10 Auscultatory areas. This shows where the valve sounds are best heard. These areas are not the surface markings of where the valves actually are (see Fig. 2.5).

aortic (second intercostal space, right sternal edge)

pulmonary area (second intercostal space, left sternal edge)

tricuspid area (left sternal edge)

mitral area (fifth intercostal space)

components of S_2 are labelled A_2P_2. P_2 is only usually heard in the pulmonary area unless it is very loud.

Occasionally, the heart sounds may be split. This is when one component of the sound occurs before the other. For example, if the mitral valve (M_1) closes before the tricuspid (T_1) then S_1 is two distinct sounds, and it is said to be split.

S_1 is usually just one sound, and it is very rarely split. Any splitting of S_1 must not be mistaken for an ejection click or even S_4 (the fourth heart sound).

S_2 is normally split on inspiration (Fig. 7.12), especially in the young. Inspiration delays right heart emptying because it causes an increased venous return. This means the pulmonary valve is open

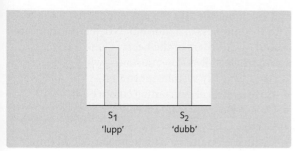

Fig. 7.11 Normal heart sound. (S_1, first heart sound; S_2, second heart sound.)

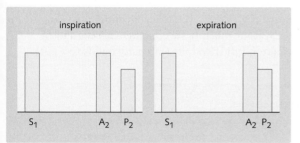

Fig. 7.12 Splitting of the second heart sound. S_2 may show physiological splitting into A_2 and P_2.

longer and so closes later. This can only be heard in the pulmonary area.

Abnormal heart sounds

The third and fourth heart sounds (S_3 and S_4, respectively) occur in diastole (Fig. 7.13), and they are caused by abnormal filling of the ventricle. S_3 is caused by passive filling in early diastole. S_4 is a consequence of atrial contraction, leading to an increased filling pressure.

S_3 is sometimes heard in healthy, young adults (younger than 35 years) and in pregnant women. Otherwise, the presence of S_3 indicates:

- Heart failure.
- Mitral regurgitation.
- Constrictive pericarditis (the high-pitched 'pericardial knock').

The presence of S_4 indicates a ventricle with increased stiffness (e.g. due to aortic stenosis or hypertension).

Clicks can be heard when abnormal aortic (e.g in aortic stenosis) or pulmonary valves open. They are called ejection systolic clicks, and they occur in early systole—it sounds as if the first heart sound is split. Similar sounds occur with abnormal mitral or tricuspid valves where the sound is mid-diastolic and called an opening snap. A prolapsed mitral valve causes midsystolic clicks.

Fig. 7.14 shows some variations of abnormal splitting in S_2.

Alterations in sound intensity can indicate disease, for example:

- S_1 is loud in mitral stenosis.
- S_1 is soft in mitral regurgitation and first-degree heart block.
- S_1 is variable in second-degree heart block and atrial fibrillation.
- A_2 is loud in systemic hypertension.
- A_2 is soft in aortic stenosis.

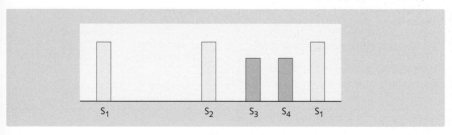

Fig. 7.13 The third and fourth heart sounds. The third heart sound creates a triple rhythm; the fourth heart sound is usually heard just before S_1 (da-lupp-dubb).

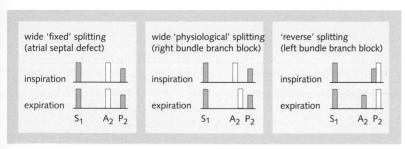

Fig. 7.14 Variations in the second heart sound. 'Fixed splitting' occurs when the second heart sound is split irrespective of respiratory movements; 'physiological splitting' refers to the normal splitting of S_2 with respiration and 'reverse splitting' occurs when the normal changes with respiration are reversed.

When listening to the heart, first concentrate on the heart sounds and establish that they are normal before attempting to listen to the murmurs.

- P_2 is loud in pulmonary hypertension.
- P_2 is soft in pulmonary stenosis.

Murmurs

Murmurs are caused by turbulent blood flow at a valve or an abnormal communication within the heart. It is customary to note the intensity of the murmur as a number out of 6 (e.g. 5/6 is a very loud murmur), but the size of a defect does not correlate with the loudness of a murmur. Not all murmurs are caused by disorders of the heart. These innocent murmurs are called flow murmurs, which typically:

- Are soft, early systolic murmurs.
- Have a musical or grunting component.
- Do not have a palpable thrill.
- Occur in the young or the elderly.
- Occur in conditions with increased blood flow (e.g. anaemia, thyrotoxicosis, hypertension, pregnancy).

Murmurs are classified according to when they are heard (i.e. systolic, diastolic, or continuous) (Fig. 7.15).

Systolic murmurs are further classified into ejection (mid) systolic (intensity builds to a peak

Classification of cardiac murmurs			
Timing	Cause	Best heard	Radiates
Systolic murmurs: Ejection systolic	Aortic stenosis	Aortic area	Neck
	Pulmonary stenosis	Left sternal edge	Loudest on inspiration
	Atrial septal defect	Left sternal edge	—
	Outflow tract obstruction	—	—
Pansystolic	Mitral regurgitation (blowing)	Apex	Axilla
	Tricuspid regurgitation (low-pitched)	Left sternal edge	—
	Ventricular septal defect (loud and rough)	Left sternal edge	—
	Mitral valve prolapse	Apex	—
Late systolic	Coarctation of aorta	Left sternal edge	—
	Hypertrophic obstructive cardiomyopathy	—	—
Diastolic murmurs: Mid-diastolic	Mitral stenosis (low rumbling)	Apex	Louder with exercise
	Tricuspid stenosis	Left sternal edge	—
	Austin–Flint	Apex	—
	Aortic regurgitation (blowing, high-pitched)	Left sternal edge	—
Early diastolic	Pulmonary regurgitation	Right sternal edge	—
	Graham–Steel in pulmonary hypertension	—	—
Continuous murmurs: Combined systolic and diastolic murmurs	Patent ductus arteriosus (machinery)	Left sternal edge	—
	Aortic stenosis and regurgitation	Left sternal edge	Neck
Venous hum	High venous flow especially in young children	Neck	Reduced while lying flat
	High mammary blood flow in a pregnant woman	—	—
Pericardial friction rub	Inflamed pericardium; scratching or crunching noise	—	Loudest in systole

Fig. 7.15 Types of cardiac murmur.

and then subsides before S_2) or pansystolic (same intensity throughout systole right up to S_2).

Murmurs are sometimes very difficult to hear when you are first starting out; it is best to try to differentiate whether the murmur is systolic or diastolic—it is most likely to be systolic. Then, try to differentiate between ejection systolic and pansystolic.

Even experts have difficulty in distinguishing some murmurs. Take every opportunity to hear as many normal hearts and obvious murmurs as possible.

In examinations where you are asked to examine the cardiovascular system, first concentrate on the chest and then inform the examiner that you would also like to examine the abdomen. Usually, the examiner will say that there is no abnormality there and not to waste your valuable time doing this examination. However, on the wards take every opportunity to examine any patient fully.

Abdomen

Inspection
Fig. 7.16 describes inspection of the abdomen for scars and skin lesions, and Fig. 7.17 shows how to tell the direction of venous flow.

Palpation
Fig. 7.18 describes palpation of the abdomen.

Percussion
Percussion can be used to outline the liver. If the liver edge cannot be felt, then percuss over the right side.

If there is dullness throughout, the liver may be so enlarged that it occupies the whole area.

Auscultation
Auscultate over the abdomen listening for bowel sounds.

If you suspect an abdominal aortic aneurysm, then auscultate over it to detect any bruits.

Inspection of the abdomen for scars and skin lesions		
Sign observed	**Test performed**	**Diagnostic inference**
Dilated veins visible	Check direction of blood flow by pressing vein and watching direction of refilling (Fig. 7.17)	If flow of blood is superior: inferior vena caval obstruction If blood flow is inferior: superior vena caval obstruction If blood flow is radiating from umbilicus: portal vein obstruction
Pulsations in the epigastric region		Abdominal aortic aneurysm; visible peristalsis

Fig. 7.16 Inspection of the abdomen for scars and skin lesions.

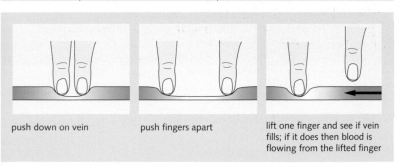

push down on vein

push fingers apart

lift one finger and see if vein fills; if it does then blood is flowing from the lifted finger

Fig. 7.17 Assessing direction of venous flow.

Fig. 7.18 Palpation of the abdomen.

Palpation of the abdomen		
Sign observed	**Test performed**	**Diagnostic inference**
Enlarged liver edge	Palpate right upper quadrant; feel liver edge by using the edge of your right hand and placing it deep; start low down and work your way up; ask the patient to breathe deeply	Right heart failure; infection; excess alcohol
Pulsatile liver edge	—	Tricuspid valve incompetence
Midline pulsatile mass	Palpate the epigastrium	Abdominal aortic aneurysm

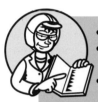

- What general points do you have to remember when taking a history?
- What are the specific points that should be covered about the presenting complaint?
- How would you take a history of a patient with a cardiovascular complaint? What specific questions would you ask?
- What signs can be seen by general inspection?
- Describe how to test for clubbing. What conditions give rise to finger clubbing?
- What are the signs of infective endocarditis?
- How would you inspect and palpate the limbs? What signs should you look for?
- Where should you palpate the peripheral pulses? How would you assess their rate and rhythm?
- What changes can occur in the pulse waveform?
- What signs of cardiovascular disease might be seen in an examination of the face?
- What changes in the retina might indicate cardiovascular disease?
- How should you view the jugular venous pulse? How does the jugular venous pressure change in disease?
- Which conditions can cause visible lesions on the chest?
- What disorders can change the apex beat?
- Describe the normal heart sounds. Are there any normal variations?
- How do we classify abnormal heart sounds? Describe how the sounds are caused. How do we describe their intensity and timing?
- Describe correct use of a stethoscope. When do you use the bell, and when the diaphragm?
- Where are the auscultatory areas of the chest? What do abnormal sounds mean in the different areas?
- Which lesions of the abdomen may have a cardiovascular cause?
- How should you palpate the abdomen when looking for an enlarged liver or aneurysm? What might cause these disorders?

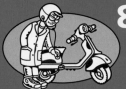

8. Investigations and Imaging

Investigation of cardiovascular function

Electrocardiography

The electrocardiogram (ECG) is a recording of the electrical activity of the heart, obtained by measuring the changes in electrical potential difference that occur on the skin. It is usually the first investigation used to diagnose arrhythmias and chest pain.

The electrical signal that activates contraction of the myocytes creates a wave of depolarization. As the wave of depolarization spreads through the ventricle there will be, at any one moment, areas of the ventricle that have been excited and areas that have not yet been excited. In effect, there is a difference in potential between them: one area is negative in charge, the other is positive. These areas can be thought of as two electrical poles. This is the cardiac dipole (Fig. 8.1). This dipole depends on both the size of the charge (which depends on the amount of muscle excited) and the direction the wave of depolarization is travelling in. Recording electrodes

are placed in certain positions on the body so that the cardiac dipole and other changes in potential can be measured in different directions.

Conventionally, the ECG is recorded using 12 leads (Fig. 8.2). Note that the term 'lead' is used to denote the direction in which the potential is measured, and not a physical electrode—only 9 electrodes are used to produce the 12 leads. The additional 3 lead traces are produced using the 'standard leads', which show the potential difference between specific pairs of unipolar leads. These leads allow us to view the electrical activity in both the frontal (I, II, III, aVR, aVL, and aVF) and transverse (V_1 to V_6) planes, and in any direction in these planes.

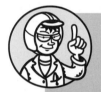

Think of depolarization as a wave on a pond that spreads out from a dropped stone. Where the muscle is narrow (e.g. the interventricular septum) imagine the wave being carried down a narrow channel.

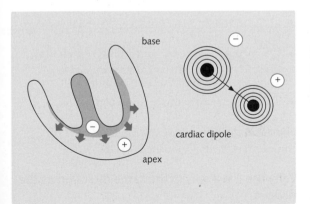

Fig. 8.1 The cardiac dipole. As the wave of depolarization travels from the atrioventricular (AV) node to the apex and base of the heart, it can be considered to move from an area of negative charge to an area of positive charge. The direction of the dipole at any time indicates how the wave of depolarization travels through the ventricle. (The area that has been excited is termed as 'negative' and the area to be excited as 'positive'. This reflects the changes in charge in the extracellular space).

Unipolar leads

Unipolar leads measure any positive potential difference directed towards their solitary electrode. These include:

- aVL, aVR, and aVF—electrodes on both arms and the left leg. They view the heart in the frontal plane.
- Six electrodes labelled V_1 to V_6—these measure any potential changes in the transverse plane, and they are arranged around the left side of the chest.

Standard leads

The potential difference shown by these leads is conventionally measured from:

- Lead I—right arm (aVR) to left arm (aVL); left arm positive.
- Lead II—right arm (aVR) to left leg (aVF); left leg positive.

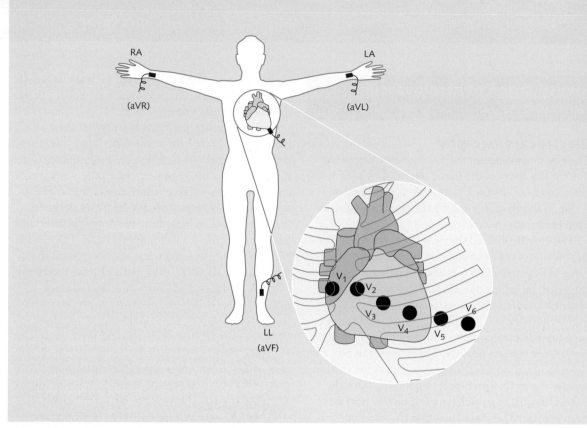

Fig. 8.2 Placement of electrocardiographic electrodes. The electrodes on the right arm (RA), left arm (LA), and left leg (LL) give the electrocardiogram trace for the frontal leads (i.e. I, II, III, aVL, aVR, and aVF). The electrodes V_1–V_6 measure the electrocardiogram in the transverse plane.

- Lead III—left arm (aVL) to left leg (aVF); left leg positive.

These bipolar limb leads view the heart in the frontal plane. These three electrodes make up Einthoven's triangle around the heart (see below).

Remember that as the dipole has both charge (amplitude) and direction, the shape of the ECG varies depending upon the position of the recording electrode. The directions measured in the frontal plane and the associated changes in the ECG trace are shown in Fig. 8.3.

Normal electrocardiogram

The classical ECG trace is shown in Fig. 8.4. The elements of an ECG are:
- P wave—due to atrial depolarization and contraction.
- PR interval—due to conduction through the atrioventricular (AV) node (approximately 120 ms).

- QRS complex—due to ventricular depolarization (approximately 80 ms).
- QT interval—due to continuing ventricular muscle depolarization (approximately 300ms).
- T wave—due to ventricular repolarization.

Note that the different components of the QRS complex are formally defined (Fig. 8.5).

Why the T wave is in the same direction as the R wave

The wave of depolarization travels from the AV node down to the apex and base of the heart. This is the cause of the R wave in the ECG. If repolarization of the heart then took place in the same direction the T wave would be in the opposite direction to the R wave. However, repolarization actually takes place from the base of the heart towards the top of the septum. Thus, the wave of repolarization is in the

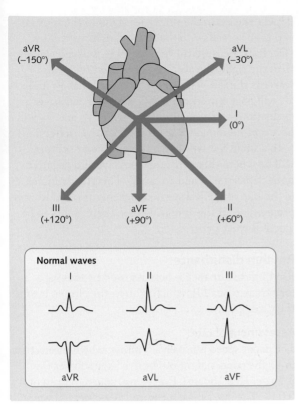

Fig. 8.3 Lead directions in the anterior plane. (Redrawn with permission from Epstein et al, eds, 1997.)

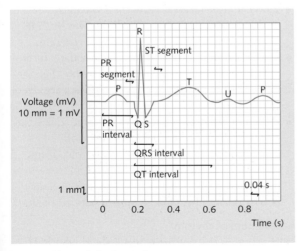

Fig. 8.4 Normal electrocardiogram.

opposite direction to the wave of depolarization, and so the T wave is upright. This is a double negative: repolarization is negative depolarization and it occurs in a negative direction, so it appears as if it is positive.

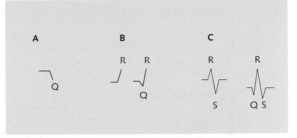

Fig. 8.5 Definitions of the ECG waves. If the wave following the P wave is negative, it is a Q wave (A). If a positive deflection follows the P wave, it is called an R wave, whether it is preceded by a Q wave or not (B). Any following negative deflection is known as an S wave, whether there has been a preceding Q wave or not (C). Abnormally large Q waves have an additional pathological significance (see Fig. 8.12).

Cardiac axis

The average direction of the wave of depolarization is the electrical axis of the heart; referred to as the cardiac axis (Fig. 8.6). It must be established whether this is normal or not. There are three ways this can be established.

When the depolarization wave in the ventricles is moving towards a lead, then the R wave will be larger than the S wave in that lead. When the ventricular depolarization wave is moving away from a lead, then the S wave will be larger than the R wave in that lead. If the S wave and R wave are equal then the depolarization is moving (on average) at right angles to that lead.

Therefore, to assess the axis, find the lead in the frontal plane with the greatest R wave. The cardiac axis is generally in this direction. Also check that the lead which measures at right angles to this has an R and S wave that are approximately equal.

An alternative method is to count the maximum height of the QRS complex in leads I and aVF and plot this point on a graph with the axes being I and aVF. Draw a line from the origin to this point. This reflects the axis of the heart (Fig. 8.6). This is an analysis of vectors with amplitude and direction (as in the parallelogram of forces). A similar approach is used when drawing Einthoven's triangle (Fig. 8.6).

The cardiac axis should be between $+90°$ and $-30°$ as shown in Fig. 8.3. Any deviation from this is abnormal and is termed right or left axis deviation.

Right axis deviation (axis more than $+90°$) is caused by:
- Right ventricular hypertrophy.
- Congenital heart disorders.

depolarization in the ventricles starts in the septum and then spreads into the left and right ventricles (Fig. 8.7). Because the left ventricle is usually larger than the right, the average depolarization heads towards the left ventricle. This means that V_1 and V_2 will have a predominant S wave (i.e. negative deflection) and a small R wave, while V_5 and V_6 will have a predominant R wave (i.e. positive deflection) with a small S wave. The interventricular septum will be where there are equal positive and negative deflections (i.e. R and S waves). This steady increase in the size of the R wave is sometimes termed R wave progression. If this is normal then there is said to be 'good' R wave progression.

Rhythm disturbance

Rhythm disturbance is best assessed by looking at a long trace of lead II, which is often the closest lead to the cardiac axis.

Assessment of rate

The paper speed is usually 25 mm/s, which means that in 1 s the paper has moved by five large squares (i.e. 0.2 s per large square). Every small square represents 0.04 s. The rate can be measured in a variety of ways:

- Divide 300 by the number of large squares between QRS complexes. That will give you a rate in beats per minute.
- Find the time interval between R waves by multiplying the number of little squares by 0.04. Divide 60 s by this time interval to give a rate.
- Find when an R wave lands on a large square. If the next R wave lands on the next large square then the rate is 300 beats/min. If it lands on the square after that then the rate is 150 beats/min, etc. (see below).
- If the interval between R waves is 1 large square the rate is 300 beats/min; 2 large squares, 150 beats/min; 3 large squares, 100 beats/min; 4 large squares, 75 beats/min; 5 large squares, 60 beats/min; 6 large squares, 50 beats/min (i.e. divide 300 by the number of large squares between beats).

Assessment of rhythm

Note whether the rhythm is regular, and whether every QRS complex is preceded by a P wave.

Note whether the PR interval is the same throughout. If the rhythm is irregular, is it irregularly irregular or regularly irregular?

Arrhythmias
Heart block

Fig. 8.8 details the electrocardiographic appearance of the heart blocks.

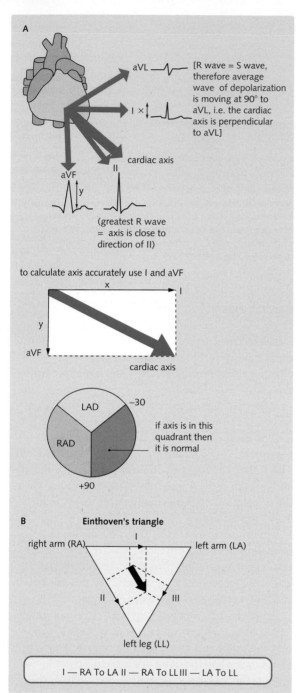

Fig. 8.6 (A) Normal axis and the different methods to measure it. (B) Einthoven's triangle. (LAD, left axis deviation; RAD, right axis deviation).

Left axis deviation (axis less than −30°) is caused by left ventricular hypertrophy.

Anterior chest leads (V_1–V_6)

The anterior chest leads look at the chest in the horizontal (or transverse) plane. The wave of

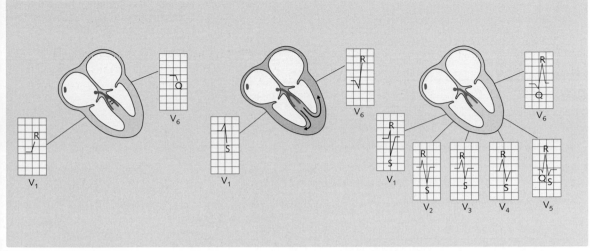

Fig. 8.7 The different anterior chest leads show different QRS traces due to the changing directions of the electrical activity. Lead V_4 is usually over the interventricular septum, and therefore usually shows equal R and S waves. Note the changing relative heights of Q, R, and S waves between leads. The changing height of the R wave from V_1 to V_6 is known as 'R wave progression'.

Bundle branch block

Delay in the conduction system of the interventricular septum leads to widening of the QRS complexes (>0.12 s) (Fig. 8.9). Looking at leads V_1 and V_6 in right bundle branch block there is:

- A second R wave (R′) in V_1 and a deeper, wider S wave in V_6.
- The last part of the QRS in lead V_1 is negative. This is because of the delayed right ventricular depolarization.

This change can also be seen in lead I, where the last part of the QRS is negative due to the delayed right ventricular depolarization.

In left bundle branch block:

- There is a Q wave with an S wave in V_1.
- There is a notched R wave in V_6.
- The last part of the QRS in lead V_1 is positive. This reflects the delayed depolarization of the left ventricle.

Again, the delayed depolarization is also reflected in lead I, where the last section of the QRS shows a positive split peak.

Atrial and ventricular rhythm disturbances

Electrocardiographic appearances of atrial and ventricular rhythm disturbances are shown in Figs 8.10 and 8.11.

Myocardial infarction

Electrocardiographic changes after myocardial infarction (Fig. 8.12) include:

- Within hours—ST elevation, and T wave lengthens and gets taller.
- Within 24 hours—T wave inversion, and ST elevation resolves.
- Within hours or days—abnormal large Q waves start to form and usually persist, T wave inversion may persist, ST segment returns to normal.

The leads in which these changes occur reflect the area of the heart affected:

- II, III, and aVF for an inferior infarct.
- V_1–V_4 for an anteroseptal infarct.
- V_4–V_6, I, and aVL for an anterolateral infarct.

In subendocardial infarction:

- There is T wave inversion.
- No Q waves form.

In true posterior infarct there is:

- A prominent R wave in V_2.
- ST depression.
- An upright T wave.

Electrocardiographic exercise test

An exercise or stress electrocardiogram is used to assess cardiac function in exercise. It is often used to

First degree block (constantly prolonged PR interval)

0.36 s

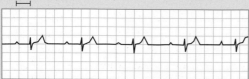

Each QRS complex has a preceding P wave, but the PR interval is 0.36 s (normal is 0.12–0.21 s), which is prolonged

Second degree block (Mobitz type II) (PR interval constant, but some P waves have no QRS)

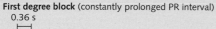

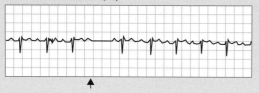

There is a constant, normal PR interval, but there are isolated P waves without following QRS complexes

Second degree block (Mobitz type I, Wenkebach) (PR interval increases with each beat and then results in an isolated P wave)

0.26 0.28 0.32 s   0.26 0.28 0.32 s

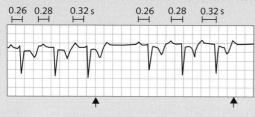

The PR interval progressively increases and then there is one isolated P wave without a following QRS complex; the PR interval then goes back to normal and starts to increase again

Second degree block (2:1 type) (every second P wave is followed by a QRS complex)

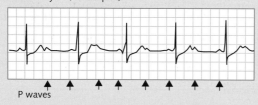

P waves

There are two P waves for every QRS complex. The PR interval of the beats with a QRS complex is normal

Third degree (complete) block (QRS complexes are independent of P waves)

P waves

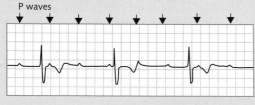

There are 90 P waves/min. There is no relationship between P waves and QRS complexes

Fig. 8.8 Classification of heart blocks. Note that only the large squares of the ECG are shown for clarity.

diagnose angina. ST depression on an exercise electrocardiogram suggests myocardial ischaemia. This may also be found in ventricular hypertrophy and abnormal ventricular conduction.

Other abnormalities

The following also affect the electrocardiogram:

- Digoxin—ST depression, T wave inversion.
- Hyperkalaemia—tall T waves, wide QRS complexes, absent P waves.
- Hypokalaemia—prolonged QT interval, small T waves, U waves (wave after T wave).
- Hypercalcaemia—short QT interval.
- Hypocalcaemia—long QT interval.

When assessing electrocardiograms, adopt the following system:

- Name, age, and sex of the patient.
- Date the electrocardiogram was taken.
- Rate.
- Rhythm.
- Axis.

Note any abnormalities and in which lead. Look at:

- P waves: width and height.
- PR interval.
- QRS complex: width and height.
- QT interval.
- ST segment.
- T waves: negative/positive and height.
- U waves.

Give a differential diagnosis.

Echocardiography

Echocardiography is increasingly used as a diagnostic technique. The echoes of ultrasound waves are used to study the heart and its function. As the ultrasound beam travels through the body, echoes are produced at tissue interfaces, and they are reflected back. Echoes from tissues furthest from the transmitter take longest to return. In this way, a picture is built up. Fluid generally shows up as black, tissues show up as white. Colour is used to indicate blood flow on machines that combine echocardiography with doppler ultrasonography (see below).

Advantages of echocardiography for cardiovascular investigation include:

- Non-invasive, painless, and harmless.
- Can be used to study the motion of the heart and valves.
- Can be used to measure velocity of blood (using the Doppler shift phenomenon) and to estimate stenosis severity from acceleration of blood through a lesion.
- Can be used to measure cardiac chamber dimensions.

Disadvantages include the fact that the ribs and lungs do not allow ultrasound to pass through them, so special sites (or windows) must be used. Most imaging is still done through the anterior chest wall, but, when necessary, an oesophageal probe can be used for transoesophageal (TOE) imaging.

Echocardiography is used to investigate:

- Valvular disease.
- Pericardial effusion.
- Aneurysms.
- Left ventricular size for a diagnosis of heart failure.

Doppler ultrasonography

This is used to measure flow in peripheral vessels. It uses ultrasound, in a similar way to that in echocardiography, to map out the vessel highlighting any stenosis.

Red blood cells move relative to the ultrasound beam. They create a Doppler shift, which is a change in the frequency of the ultrasound echo that returns to the transducer. The shift in frequency is directly proportional to the velocity of the blood.

Colour can be used to differentiate blood flowing towards the probe from blood flowing away. It is commonly used to assess peripheral vessel function before angiography.

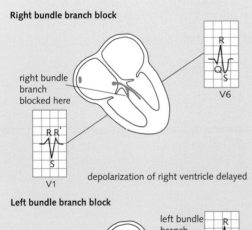

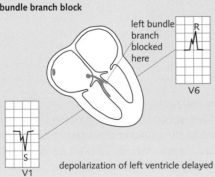

Right bundle branch block

right bundle branch blocked here

V6

V1

depolarization of right ventricle delayed

Left bundle branch block

left bundle branch blocked here

V6

V1

depolarization of left ventricle delayed

Fig. 8.9 Left and right bundle branch blocks. Disruption of the conduction system delays activation of ventricular muscle producing a characteristic split peak in the ECG.

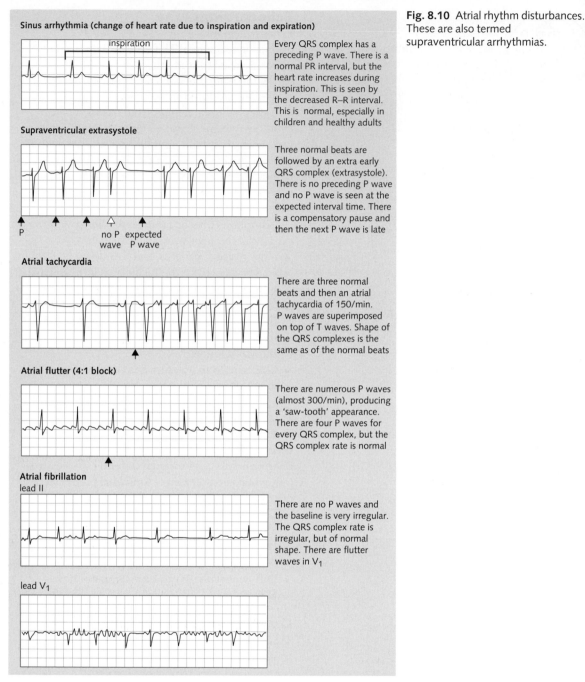

Sinus arrhythmia (change of heart rate due to inspiration and expiration)

inspiration

Every QRS complex has a preceding P wave. There is a normal PR interval, but the heart rate increases during inspiration. This is seen by the decreased R–R interval. This is normal, especially in children and healthy adults

Supraventricular extrasystole

P / no P / expected / wave / P wave

Three normal beats are followed by an extra early QRS complex (extrasystole). There is no preceding P wave and no P wave is seen at the expected interval time. There is a compensatory pause and then the next P wave is late

Atrial tachycardia

There are three normal beats and then an atrial tachycardia of 150/min. P waves are superimposed on top of T waves. Shape of the QRS complexes is the same as of the normal beats

Atrial flutter (4:1 block)

There are numerous P waves (almost 300/min), producing a 'saw-tooth' appearance. There are four P waves for every QRS complex, but the QRS complex rate is normal

Atrial fibrillation
lead II

There are no P waves and the baseline is very irregular. The QRS complex rate is irregular, but of normal shape. There are flutter waves in V_1

lead V_1

Fig. 8.10 Atrial rhythm disturbances. These are also termed supraventricular arrhythmias.

Cardiac catheterization

Originally performed to directly measure the pressures in the right heart, left ventricle, aorta, and pulmonary artery in patients with valvular disease, catheterization is now primarily used for angiography (see below). Echocardiography is now the method of choice to assess valvular function.

A thin radio-opaque catheter is introduced into the circulation and advanced towards the heart using occasional radiographs or fluoroscopy. The right heart is reached through a peripheral vein and by threading the catheter through the right atrium and into the right ventricle. The left heart is reached by a catheter entered through a peripheral artery and advanced through the aorta and the aortic valve into the left ventricle.

To produce an angiogram, the catheter is used to inject a radio-opaque contrast medium into the heart

Fig. 8.11 Ventricular rhythm disturbances.

Ventricular extrasystole (extraventricular beat)

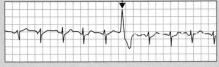

There are five sinus beats and then a ventricular extrasystole occurs, which is a wide QRS complex with an abnormal T wave.

Ventricular extrasystole with R on T phenomenon

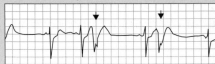

In this phenomenon the extrasystole beats occur on the T wave of the previous beat. It is said to be an 'R on T' phenomenon (i.e. an R wave on top of a T wave).

Ventricular tachycardia

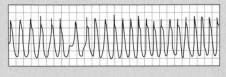

The rate of QRS complexes is almost 300/min. The QRS complexes are wide and abnormal in shape. There are no preceding P waves. This can often lead to ventricular fibrillation.

Paroxysmal tachycardia (sometimes called junctional tachycardia)

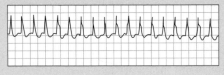

Rate is increased at 200/min, but there are preceding P waves and normal-shaped QRS complexes, which are slightly wider than normal due to a rate-related bundle branch block. This is due to re-entry in the AV node or an accessory pathway (e.g. Wolff–Parkinson–White).

Ventricular fibrillation

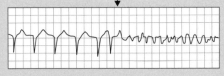

This occurs after the five QRS complexes. There are no QRS complexes, the baseline wanders, and there is no regularity to the ECG. The ventricular wall is fibrillating and there is no organized contraction. Immediate intervention is necessary as death is imminent.

Asystole

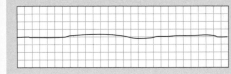

There is an absence of any heart contraction and there are no complexes in the ECG. The baseline is seen to wander slightly, but is essentially flat.

or vessels. Angiograms are especially useful for viewing the coronary arteries for any stenosis. They are often performed before angioplasty or coronary artery bypass graft operations. Peripheral arteries can also be viewed with a similar process with the catheter being guided to the arterial tree to be viewed.

If right heart catheterization is performed, blood samples can also be taken to measure levels of local metabolites in the heart. Congenital shunts can be estimated from measurements of oxygen saturation at different sites in the heart. Cardiac output can also be measured by thermodilution.

Nuclear cardiology
Nuclear cardiology is used to look at myocardial function, especially in ischaemia. It uses

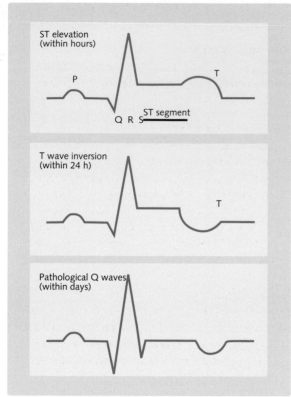

Fig. 8.12 ST elevation, T wave inversion, and Q waves after a myocardial infarction. Abnormal Q waves result from an electrode over an area of full thickness infarction.

radioisotopes, which emit radioactive particles that can be detected when they decay.

Different radioisotopes have different affinities for various tissues; for example, thallium–201 is taken up by healthy myocardium, but not by ischaemic myocardium, thereby mapping the ischaemic area as a cold spot.

The technique can be used for subjects at rest and during exercise.

Commonly used methods in nuclear cardiology are:
- Thallium-201 imaging—to assess myocardial perfusion before and after exercise. It is used to detect ischaemia and infarction.
- Radionuclide ventriculography—uses blood labelled with technetium-99m to assess ventricular structure and function. Ventricular diastolic and systolic volumes are measured, which can be used to calculate the ejection fraction.

Note that techniques using magnetic resonance imaging for similar testing are under development (see below).

Pulmonary investigation

The pulmonary circulation can be investigated using ventilation/perfusion (V/Q) tests, which check for mismatches between air entry and the supply of blood to the alveoli (fully described in *Crash Course: Respiratory System*). More invasive tests include pulmonary angiography, particularly when pulmonary emboli are suspected.

Biochemical markers of myocardial damage

Cellular enzymes and other intracellular proteins are released by necrotic tissue. Testing for the proteins specifically released from cardiac tissues can be a useful aid in confirming myocardial infarction (Fig. 8.13). The enzymes tested for include creatine kinase (CK), aspartate aminotransferase (AST), and lactate dehydrogenase (LDH), although tests for the classic cardiac enzymes have largely been replaced by measurement of troponin T (Tn-T) or troponin I (Tn-I), regulatory proteins on thin filaments, which leak from damaged myocytes. Tn-T levels peak 12–24 hours after myocardial injury, but may remain elevated for over a week. Elevated plasma Tn-T is both very sensitive and very specific for cardiac damage, but episodes of reversible ischaemia may also elevate plasma troponin levels. Current guidelines are that a peak plasma Tn-T between 0.1 and 0.2 ng/mL indicates unstable angina, with a peak plasma Tn-T>0.2 ng/mL indicating myocardial infarction.

Myoglobin, a protein that aids the transport of oxygen in the cells, is also sometimes used. This peaks at 2–4 hours and may persist for several days.

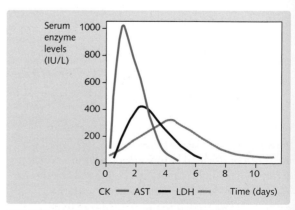

Fig. 8.13 Levels of classic cardiac enzymes after myocardial infarction. (CK, creatine kinase; AST, aspartate aminotransferase; LDH, lactate dehydrogenase.) (Redrawn with permission from Forbes and Jackson, 1993.)

Creatine kinase

Creatine kinase peaks within 24 hours of infarction, and it returns to normal within 2 days. It is also produced by skeletal muscle and brain, so the isoenzyme specific to myocardium (CK–MB) is also sometimes measured. The level of enzyme released directly relates to the size of the infarction.

Creatine kinase levels can also be increased as a result of an intramuscular injection or the patient falling.

This enzyme is usually used to confirm a diagnosis of myocardial infarction.

Aspartate aminotransferase

Aspartate aminotransferase peaks after 1–2 days, and it returns to normal within 3 days. It is also produced from liver, kidney, lungs, and red blood cells.

Lactate dehydrogenase

Lactate dehydrogenase peaks after 2–3 days, and it stays high for 1 week. It is also released from skeletal muscle, liver, and red blood cells. LDH-1—also known as hydroxybutyrate dehydrogenase (HBD)—is the most cardiospecific of the five isoenzymes of lactate dehydrogenase. Lactate dehydrogenase is often used for a retrospective diagnosis of myocardial infarction.

Routine investigations

Haematology

Fig. 8.14 outlines the tests that can be performed when assessing haematological problems in the cardiovascular system.

Clinical chemistry

Fig. 8.15 outlines the clinical chemistry tests that can be performed when assessing the cardiovascular system. Much biochemical data cannot be looked at individually (e.g. in dehydration there will probably be an increased concentration of sodium, potassium, chloride, etc.). Usually these tests are performed using blood, but urine can also be tested (e.g. for protein, glucose).

Microbiology

Any sample of the body can be sent for cell culture and sensitivity testing. The microbiology department will attempt to grow any microorganisms present (culture) and determine what antibiotics can be used in treatment (sensitivity).

Viral serology may help to diagnose acute myocarditis (coxsackievirus). Samples sent are usually blood or sputum. Blood is indicated for

Normal values for clinical haematology			
Component	Normal range	Change from normal	Reason
Haemoglobin	Male: 13–17 g/dL	High	Polycythaemia
	Female: 12–15 g/dL	Low	Anaemia
Red blood cells	Male: $4.4–5.8 \times 10^{12}$/L	High	Polycythaemia
	Female: $4.0–5.2 \times 10^{12}$/L	Low	Anaemia
White blood cells	$4–10 \times 10^9$/L	High	Infection, trauma, haemorrhage, inflammation, infarction
		Low	Infection, corticosteroid therapy
Platelet count	$150–400 \times 10^9$/L	High	Thrombocythaemia
		Low	Thrombocytopenia
Erythrocyte sedimentation rate (ESR)	Male: < age in years/2 Female: < (age in years + 10)/2	High: non-specific indication of disease	Myocardial infarction, vasculitis, systemic lupus erythematosus, rheumatoid arthritis, malignancy

Fig. 8.14 Normal values for clinical haematology.

Normal values in clinical chemistry			
Substance analysed	Normal range	Change from normal	Causes
Electrolytes Urea	3.3–6.7 mmol/L	High	Renal failure
Creatinine	60–120 µmol/L	High	Renal failure
Na^+	135–145 mmol/L	High Low	Dehydration, hyperaldosteronism Diuretics, aldosterone deficiency, water excess
K^+	3.6–5.0 mmol/L	High or low	Can lead to arrhythmias
Cl^-	103–110 mmol/L	—	—
Ca^{2+}	2.2–2.6 mmol/L	High Low	Malignancy; thiazide diuretics; thyrotoxicosis Renal failure; blood transfusion
HCO_3^-	24–30 mmol/L	High Low	Metabolic/respiratory alkalosis Metabolic/respiratory acidosis
Glucose (fasting)	2.8–6.0 mmol/L	High	Impaired glucose tolerance
pO_2 (arterial)	11–15 kPa (85–105 mmHg)	Low	Respiratory failure Hyperventilation
pCO_2 (arterial)	4.5–6.0 kPa (35–46 mmHg)	Low High	Respiratory failure
Thyroid function TSH T_4 T_3	0.3–0.4 mU/L 9–26 pmol/L 3–8.8 pmol/L	High TSH, low T_4, T_3 Low TSH, high T_4, T_3	Hypothyroidism Hyperthyroidism
Cholesterol: total	<5.2 mmol/L	High	Hypercholesterolaemia (may be familial)
High-density lipoprotein	>1.2 mmol/L	Low	Predisposes to atherosclerosis
Low-density lipoprotein	<3.5 mmol/L	High	Hypercholesterolaemia (may be familial)
Triglyceride (fasting)	0.4–1.8 mmol/L	High	Hyperlipidaemia
Osmolality	280–295 mmol/L	High Low	Dehydration Water overload

Fig. 8.15 Normal values in clinical chemistry. (T_3, tri-iodothyronine; T_4, thyroxine; TSH, thyroid stimulating hormone.)

suspected cases of infective endocarditis (*Streptococcus viridans*) and rheumatic fever (*Streptococcus pyogenes*). Sputum is indicated for suspected cases of tuberculosis (*Mycobacterium tuberculosis*).

Frequently an abnormality in one investigation is not diagnostic of a condition. You must look at various factors to reach a definite diagnosis. For example, a raised ESR and white cell count may indicate infection, but this can only be proved by a positive culture or serological test.

Histopathology

Usually, samples sent for histopathological diagnosis are biopsies of the lesion. It is most commonly used for the following:

- Vasculitis—polyarteritis nodosa, Wegener's granulomatosis, and Takayasu's arteritis.
- Cardiac tumours—atrial myxoma.
- Vascular tumours—haemangiomas.

Imaging of the cardiovascular system

Radiography
Plain radiography
Examples of plain chest radiographs are shown in Figs 8.16–8.19.

Fig. 8.16 shows a normal posteroanterior (PA) chest radiograph. The width of the heart shadow is less than half of the transthoracic diameter. Note that it is only possible to comment on the heart size on the PA radiograph and not on an anteroposterior (AP) view.

A normal lateral chest radiograph is shown in Fig. 8.17. This is a useful view, especially if an abnormality is seen on the PA chest radiograph. It helps to localize any lesions. For example, left atrial enlargement is seen as a posterior projection indenting the oesophagus. Fig. 8.18 shows an aneurysm of the left ventricle. Fig. 8.19 shows heart failure, with early pulmonary congestion.

Angiography

Fig. 8.20 shows examples of normal right and left pulmonary angiograms, while an example of pulmonary embolism of the right and left lobe is shown in Fig. 8.21.

Ultrasound
Echocardiography

A parasternal long axis view is shown in Fig. 8.22, while intracardiac thrombus is shown in Fig. 8.23, and mitral stenosis in Fig. 8.24.

A good system for looking at radiographs is as follows:
- Name, age, and sex of patient.
- Date radiograph was taken.
- Is it AP (anteroposterior) or PA (posteroanterior)?
- Is it erect or supine?
- What is the penetration like (are the vertebral bodies just visible under the heart)?
- Is there any rotation (are the clavicles symmetrical)?
- Describe any abnormalities in:
  - Mediastinum.
  - Cardiac shadow.
  - Lung fields.
  - Ribs.
  - Diaphragm.
- Suggest a differential diagnosis.

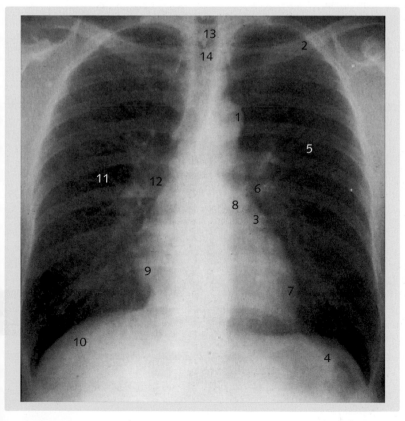

Fig. 8.16 Normal posteroanterior (PA) chest radiograph. (Courtesy of Professor Dame M Turner-Warwick, Dr M Hodson, Professor B Corrin, and Dr I Kerr.)

 1 arch of aorta/aortic knuckle
 2 clavicle
 3 left atrial appendage
 4 left dome of diaphragm
 5 left lung
 6 left hilum
 7 left ventricular border
 8 pulmonary trunk
 9 right atrial border
10 right dome of diaphragm
11 right lung
12 right hilum
13 spine of vertebrae
14 trachea

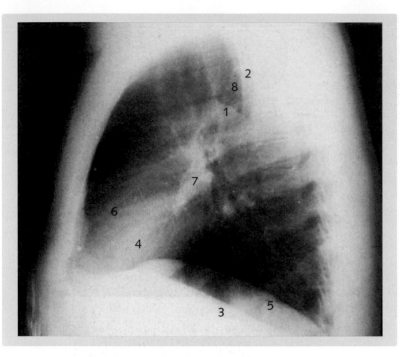

Fig. 8.17 Normal lateral chest radiograph. (Courtesy of Professor Dame M Turner-Warwick, Dr M Hodson, Professor B Corrin, and Dr I Kerr.)
1 aortic arch
2 anterior borders of scapulae
3 left dome of diaphragm
4 left ventricle
5 right dome of diaphragm
6 right ventricle
7 left atrium
8 trachea

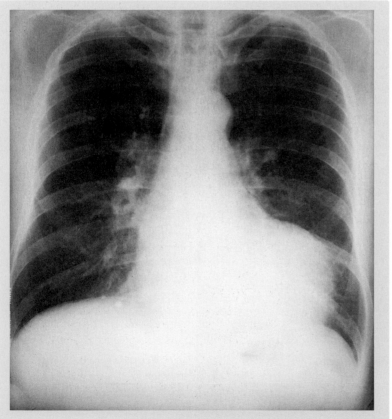

Fig. 8.18 Radiograph of an aneurysm of the left ventricle. This is a rare source of arterial embolism, which may occur some months after a myocardial infarct. Note the large heart shadow and how it occupies more than half of the transthoracic diameter. Contrast the normal appearance of the lung fields here with the congested fields in Fig. 8.19. (Courtesy of Professor JJF Belch, Mr PT McCollum, Mr PA Stonebridge, and Professor WF Walker.)

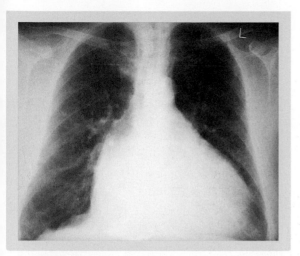

Fig. 8.19 Radiograph of the chest showing early pulmonary congestion. Note that the width of the heart shadow is greater than half the transthoracic diameter and that there are distended hila with increased lung markings. This indicates heart failure and pulmonary congestion. (Courtesy of Dr A Timmis and Dr S Brecker.)

Tomography
Computerized tomography (CT)

An example of an aortic aneurysm is shown in Fig. 8.25.

This imaging modality enables precise measurement of the size of the aneurysm. The whole body is imaged as slices or sections using X-rays. It can be used to produce a three-dimensional image, and it may also be used to perform angiography using radio-opaque contrast medium.

Magnetic resonance imaging (MRI)

MRI of the chest enables an accurate assessment to be made of the dimensions of the heart walls and lumen. Fig. 8.26 shows a normal coronal view of the chest, while Fig. 8.27 shows an extensive aortic dissection.

MRI allows better visualization of soft tissue than CT. It is safer than CT as it does not involve harmful radiation. MRI may also be set to show moving blood, to produce an image similar to an angiogram. This has replaced conventional angiography for peripheral arteries, where MRI is available. Heart movement currently restricts the visualization of the coronary arteries to the large proximal vessels only.

The use of gadolinium as a contrast agent allows delineation of perfused myocardium during the

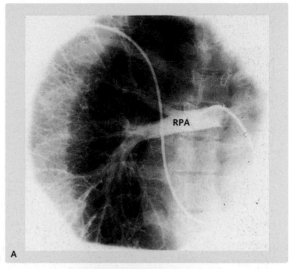

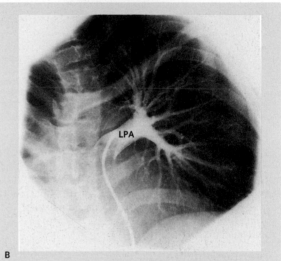

Fig. 8.20 Normal right (A) and left (B) pulmonary angiograms. The contrast agent highlights the entire arterial tree from the right and left pulmonary arteries. (LPA, left pulmonary artery; RPA, right pulmonary artery.) (Courtesy of Dr A Timmis and Dr S Brecker.)

first pass and of infarcted tissue 15–20 minutes later.

Nuclear imaging

Fig. 8.28 shows nuclear tomograms after injection of ^{99m}Tc-labelled methoxy-isobutyl-isonitrile (MIBI), demonstrating myocardial perfusion. Isotope is distributed homogeneously throughout the left ventricular myocardium, at rest and on exercise, reflecting normal myocardial perfusion.

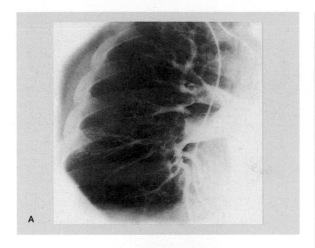

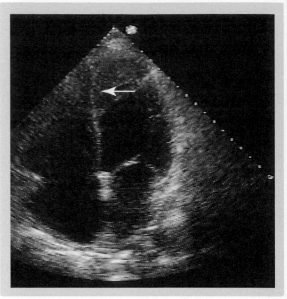

Fig. 8.23 Echocardiogram of an intracardiac thrombus. Here, layered thrombus (arrowed) is shown at the cardiac apex in relation to a previous myocardial infarct. (Courtesy of Dr A Timmis and Dr S Brecker.)

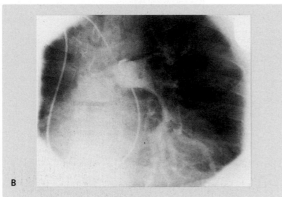

Fig. 8.21 Pulmonary angiograms showing pulmonary embolism of the right lung (A) and left lung (B). Contrast agent does not reach the distal part of the arterial tree, implying that there is some blockage. (Courtesy of Dr A Timmis and Dr S Brecker.)

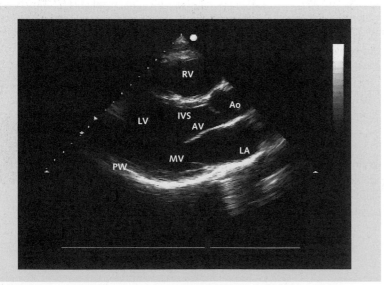

Fig. 8.22 Echocardiogram of the parasternal long axis view (diastolic frame). (Ao, aorta; AV, aortic valve; IVS, intraventricular septum; LA, left atrium; LV, left ventricle; MV, mitral valve; PW, posterior LV wall; RV, right ventricle.) (Courtesy of Dr A Timmis and Dr S Brecker.)

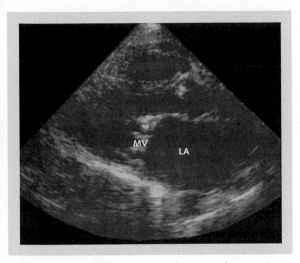

Fig. 8.24 Echocardiogram of mitral stenosis (long axis). The mitral valve (MV) leaflets are densely thickened and the left atrium (LA) is severely dilated. (Courtesy of Dr A Timmis and Dr S Brecker.)

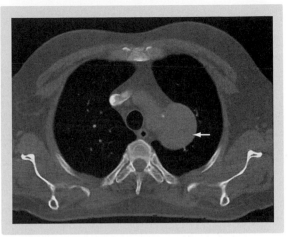

Fig. 8.25 CT of a thoracic aortic aneurysm. The scan shows a large aneurysm of the descending aortic arch (arrowed) arising just after the left subclavian branch. This is the typical location for dissecting aortic aneurysms although a dissection cannot be seen in this film. (Courtesy of Dr A Timmis and Dr S Brecker.)

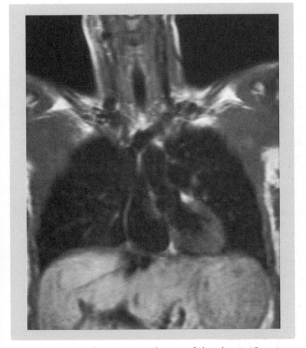

Fig. 8.26 Normal MRI coronal view of the chest. (Courtesy of Dr A Timmis and Dr S Brecker.)

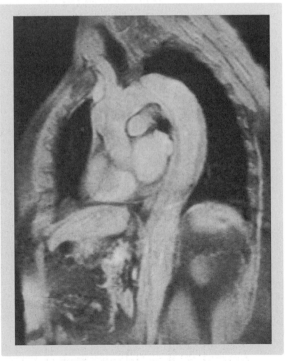

Fig. 8.27 Sagittal MRI scan showing extensive aortic dissection. Note how the descending aorta seems to have two lumens (double-barrelled). (Courtesy of Dr A Timmis and Dr S Brecker.)

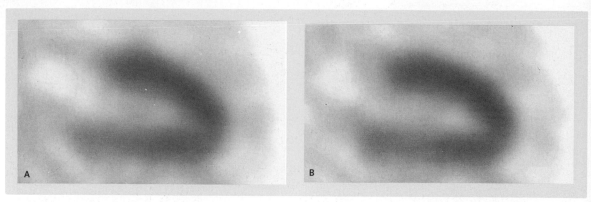

Fig. 8.28 Nuclear tomograms at rest (A) and during exercise (B) after injection of ^{99m}Tc-labelled MIBI, demonstrating myocardial perfusion. The example shown here is a vertical long axis view. (Courtesy of Dr A Timmis and Dr S Brecker.)

- What does the ECG measure?
- What is the cardiac dipole? How does it arise?
- What is the difference between a lead and an electrode? What are the two different kinds of lead?
- Where would you place electrocardiograph electrodes?
- Sketch a 'typical' ECG trace, showing the normal wave and normal parameters.
- How do you determine the cardiac axis?
- How does the ECG trace change across the anterior chest leads? Do any have a special location, and what can you learn from looking at the trace across all 6?
- What are the major types of arrhythmia?
- Describe how the electrocardiogram changes in these arrhythmias.
- What electrocardiographic changes occur in myocardial infarction?
- When would you use echocardiography? What would you be looking for?
- What is the major role of cardiac catheterization?
- Explain what the 'Doppler shift' is. How is it useful?
- Describe how cardiac enzyme levels in blood change after a myocardial infarction.
- What are the normal values for haemoglobin, white blood cells, and ESR?
- What decreases haemoglobin levels, and what can increase the ESR?
- Which electrolytes are usually measured? What are their normal levels?
- Describe how you would view a plain radiograph.
- What is the basis for thallium imaging in nuclear cardiology?
- How would you interpret other images of the cardiovascular system?

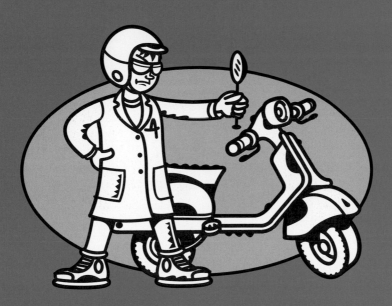

SELF-ASSESSMENT

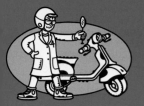

Multiple-choice Questions

Indicate whether each answer is true or false.

Chapter 1—Overview of the Cardiovascular System

1. Functions of the cardiovascular system include:

(a) Transport of nutrients.
(b) Hormonal control.
(c) Host defence.
(d) Temperature regulation.
(e) Reproduction.

Chapter 2—Structure and Function of the Heart

2. In a normal heart:

(a) A branch of the right coronary artery supplies the AV node.
(b) Aortic valves receive their blood supply from the vasa vasorum of the aorta.
(c) Conduction velocity through the AV node is relatively fast.
(d) Adrenaline acts on β_2-receptors causing coronary artery dilatation.
(e) The atrial myocardium secretes atrial natriuretic peptide in response to stretch.

3. In cardiac myocytes:

(a) Myocyte resting membrane potential is –90 mV.
(b) Positive inotropes act by reducing intracellular Ca^{2+}.
(c) Gap junctions hold myocytes together at branch points.
(d) Nodal, Purkinje fibre, and contractile (work) cells are all myocytes.
(e) The pacemaker potential decays partly due to inward leakage of Na^+.

4. The adult heart:

(a) Is related posteriorly to the oesophagus, left main bronchus, and aorta.
(b) Has a diaphragmatic surface formed mainly by the right ventricle.
(c) Has the right ventricle forming most of its inferior border.
(d) Is totally enclosed by serous pericardium.
(e) Has a fossa ovalis in the atrioventricular wall of the right atrium.

5. Regarding the structure of the heart:

(a) The aortic valve is bicuspid.
(b) The fibrous skeleton normally allows only one route of electrical conduction.
(c) The right atrium has four openings for pulmonary arteries.
(d) Papillary muscles are required for atrioventricular valve function.
(e) All venous drainage passes through the coronary sinus.

6. The normal action potential:

(a) Is dependent on cytoplasmic and extracellular Na^+ and K^+ ionic concentration differences.
(b) The resting myocyte membrane is most permeable to K^+.
(c) In nodal cells, Na^+ is responsible for a fast upstroke.
(d) The Nernst equation predicts ionic membrane permeability.
(e) The fast upstroke in contractile cells is mediated by K^+.

7. Regarding excitation–contraction coupling:

(a) Cytoplasmic $Ca2^+$ influx couples excitation and contraction.
(b) The increased force of contraction associated with an increased heart rate is known as the Treppe effect.
(c) Produces tension proportional to the level of Ca^{2+}.
(d) Changes in contractility are mediated by changes in Ca^{2+} concentration.
(e) Positive chronotropes increase the strength of contraction.

8. Concerning the embryological development of the heart:

(a) The heart only starts developing at 6 weeks gestation.
(b) The atria are separated by the septum spurium.
(c) The truncus arteriosus rotates to align itself with the ventricles.
(d) The ventricular septum has a membranous part superior to a muscular section.
(e) The left atrium initially starts with only one pulmonary vein.

9. The myocardium:

(a) Has a thick fibrous epicardium directly in contact with it.
(b) Has an endothelial layer lining its inner surface.
(c) Consists solely of cardiac work myocytes and nodal cells.
(d) Only differs from skeletal muscle in that it has a diad T-tubule system.
(e) Must function together for it to maintain function.

10. Regarding the electrical activity of the heart:

(a) The ventricular action potential lasts about 0.3 s.
(b) The upstroke in the ventricular action potential is due to the opening of potassium channels.
(c) The sinoatrial node generates more frequent action potentials than the atrioventricular node.

(d) Purkinje cells form the slowest conduction fibres.

(e) The action potential lasts as long as the contraction—this is why cardiac cells do not tetanize.

11. In the cardiac cycle:

(a) In each beat, the left ventricle ejects more blood than the right ventricle.

(b) The mitral valve opens when the left atrial pressure is greater than the left ventricular pressure.

(c) The first heart sound occurs at the end of isovolumetric contraction.

(d) Isovolumetric means 'without changing volume'.

(e) Atrial contraction is essential for ventricular filling.

12. In the electrocardiogram:

(a) The Q wave is caused by atrial repolarization.

(b) The PR interval is prolonged in atrial hypertrophy.

(c) The QT interval will give you the duration of ventricular systole.

(d) The first heart sound occurs at the same time as the P wave.

(e) The R wave coincides with the depolarization of the apex.

13. In a normal subject:

(a) Cardiac output is affected by central venous pressure, contractility, and total peripheral resistance.

(b) The end-diastolic pressure gives an indication of the size of the ventricle at the beginning of systole.

(c) Cardiac output would fall if the vagal nerves were cut.

(d) Starling's curve shifts depending on the heart's contractility.

(e) Cardiac output can only double in exercise.

14. The following are true for Starling's law:

(a) The force of contraction is inversely proportional to the initial length of the cardiac muscle fibre.

(b) The law is only true for isolated heart–lung preparations.

(c) The law means that the stroke volume is proportional to end-diastolic volume unless the contractility or vascular resistance change.

(d) As a consequence of the law, factors that reduce cardiac filling will increase contractility.

(e) The law is dependent on the integrity of the cardiac stretch receptors.

15. In the normal heart:

(a) Cardiac output is the product of heart rate and end-diastolic volume.

(b) Contractility is defined as the force of contraction for a given fibre length.

(c) End-diastolic volume and end-diastolic pressure are closely related.

(d) The Starling curve peaks and turns down due to overstretch of individual myocytes.

(e) Total peripheral resistance is defined as arterial pressure divided by cardiac output.

Chapter 3—Structure and Function of the Vessels

16. Regarding regulation of smooth muscle cell tension:

(a) EDRF requires cGMP to produce relaxation.

(b) Adrenaline requires cAMP to produce vasodilatation.

(c) Sympathetic innervation of smooth muscle uses noradrenaline.

(d) Hypoxia produces relaxation through hyperpolarization of the membrane.

(e) Tension in smooth muscle requires as much energy to maintain as in skeletal muscle.

17. Regarding capillary transport:

(a) Hydrostatic pressure is higher at the venous capillary end.

(b) There is a net effusion from the capillaries.

(c) Significant amounts of metabolites are transported by capillary fluid effusion.

(d) Hypoalbuminaemia will increase net fluid filtration out from the capillaries.

(e) Diffusion of metabolites occurs through endothelial cells (EC) and between them.

18. At birth:

(a) Pulmonary vascular resistance falls rapidly.

(b) After birth, the atrial pressures are equal.

(c) Prostaglandins are involved in maintaining the patency of the ductus venosus.

(d) The ductus arteriosus closes soon after birth due to reverse flow from the aorta.

(e) The septum primum closes the foramen ovale.

19. Vascular resistance:

(a) Is determined principally by vessel lumenal diameter.

(b) Is low in capillaries because of a large total cross-sectional area.

(c) Is important in determining blood pressure.

(d) Follows Laplace's law.

(e) Does not vary with length.

20. The vasculature:

(a) Consists of conductance, resistance, and capacitance vessels.

(b) Has arteries, which have more muscular and elastic walls than veins.

(c) Has large arteries as its main resistance vessels.

(d) Is supplied solely by blood that is in the lumen of its vessels.

(e) Functions mainly to supply cells with nutrients and remove metabolites.

21. In normal vessels:

(a) The endothelium provides a friction-free surface for blood flow.

(b) The endothelium secretes many hormones, which have systemic actions.

(c) Vascular smooth muscle contracts under sympathetic stimulation.
(d) Nitric oxide also causes smooth muscle contraction.
(e) Ca^{2+} ions play a vital role in the excitation–contraction coupling.

22. Flow through blood vessels:

(a) Varies with the pressure difference between one end and the other.
(b) Is directly proportional to the square of the radius.
(c) Increases directly with the length of the vessel.
(d) Varies inversely with the viscosity of the blood.
(e) Is directly proportional to the velocity of the blood.

23. Capillaries:

(a) Contain, at any one time, 50% of the blood volume.
(b) Have a diameter that is about the same as that of a red blood cell.
(c) Have precapillary sphincters of smooth muscle.
(d) Allow lipid-soluble substances to directly cross their walls.
(e) Control vascular resistance by constricting their walls.

24. Lymphatics:

(a) Drain excess filtrate from the interstitium.
(b) Return lymph to the subclavian artery.
(c) Play a role in the immune response by transferring antigen to lymph nodes.
(d) Are the main transport of protein from the gut.
(e) Are very extensive in the brain.

25. Major branches of the aorta include:

(a) Renal arteries.
(b) Internal iliac artery.
(c) Right brachial artery.
(d) Left colic artery.
(e) Inferior mesenteric artery.

26. Regarding the innervation of the cardiovascular system:

(a) The vagus nerve innervates the sinoatrial and atrioventricular nodes.
(b) The atria, ventricles, and conducting system receive sympathetic innervation.
(c) β_1 receptors predominate in vascular smooth muscle.
(d) Cholinergic nerves innervate the ventricular myocardium via M2 muscarinic receptors.
(e) Under normal conditions, vagal inhibition is stronger than sympathetic stimulation.

Chapter 4—Control of the Cardiovascular System

27. Regarding regulation of blood flow:

(a) Nitric oxide mediates the response to hypoxia.
(b) Autoregulation describes the regulation of blood flow in response to blood pressure changes.
(c) Hyperaemia is a pathological increase in blood flow.

(d) Increased sympathetic activity produces only vasoconstriction.
(e) Increased parasympathetic activity leads solely to vasodilatation.

28. Regarding hormonal control:

(a) Renin is released from stromal cells in the kidney.
(b) Brain natriuretic peptide is released from the ventricles in response to stretch.
(c) Vasopressin is released from the hypothalamus in response to osmolarity changes.
(d) Angiotensin I acts on smooth muscle to produce vasoconstriction.
(e) Aldosterone increases Na^+ and water retention.

29. Myogenic autoregulation:

(a) Keeps blood flow constant despite changes in mean arterial blood pressure.
(b) Is caused by contraction of smooth muscle induced by stretch.
(c) Keeps blood flow constant regardless of metabolic activity.
(d) Is dependent on neuronal innervation.
(e) Is unaffected by hypoxia.

30. If blood pressure falls, reflex effects mediated by baroreceptors include:

(a) Constriction of cerebral arterioles.
(b) Constriction of skeletal muscle arterioles.
(c) Constriction of veins.
(d) Decrease in ventilation.
(e) Increase in force of cardiac contraction.

31. Concerning regional blood flow:

(a) Blood flow to the skin increases during heavy exercise.
(b) Blood flow to the myocardium increases when the heart rate increases.
(c) The pulmonary vessels contain about one third of the blood volume at any one time.
(d) Cerebral blood flow varies little in normal circumstances.
(e) Blood flow to the kidneys is high relative to their oxygen requirement.

32. During prolonged exercise the following take place:

(a) Muscle blood flow increases because of increased parasympathetic vasodilatation.
(b) Cardiac output increases because of the Starling mechanism.
(c) Muscle blood flow increases partly due to the action of local metabolites.
(d) Blood flow to the skin increases to increase heat loss.
(e) The stroke volume may increase tenfold.

33. The cardiovascular response to training includes:

(a) Thickening of the ventricular wall.
(b) Increased vascularization of the myocardium.

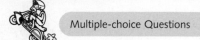
(c) Increased haemoglobin levels.
(d) Increased vascularization of skeletal muscle.
(e) An increased maximum heart rate.

34. Changes on standing:

(a) Are known as orthostasis.
(b) Involve the baroreceptors.
(c) Act to counter the effects of gravity.
(d) Include peripheral vasodilatation.
(e) Act to preserve cerebral blood flow.

Chapter 5—The Cardiovascular System in Disease

35. Features of cardiac failure include:

(a) Tiredness.
(b) Breathlessness.
(c) Nocturnal cough.
(d) Enlarged liver.
(e) Haemoptysis.

36. A ventricular rather than superventricular tachycardia is suggested by:

(a) A ventricular rate >160 beats per minute.
(b) Termination of arrhythmia with carotid sinus pressure.
(c) Variable intensity of the first heart sound.
(d) The presence of cardiac failure.
(e) QRS complexes <0.14 s in length on an ECG.

37. Regarding cardiac rhythms:

(a) Supraventricular rhythms originate in the atrioventricular node.
(b) A normal rate is between 40 and 120 beats per minute.
(c) Sinus arrhythmia is normal.
(d) Tachycardia or atrial fibrillation frequently occur in Wolff–Parkinson–White syndrome.
(e) The PR interval is increased with first degree heart block.

38. Atrial fibrillation is:

(a) Associated with an irregularly irregular pulse.
(b) Present in 10% of the elderly over 75 years.
(c) Amenable to treatment with DC cardioversion.
(d) A recognized result of thyrotoxicosis.
(e) Incompatible with life.

39. Amiodarone may cause:

(a) Pulmonary alveolitis.
(b) Liver damage.
(c) Constipation.
(d) Asthma.
(e) Thyroid disorders.

40. Angiotensin-converting enzyme inhibitors:

(a) Act mainly on enzymes in the lung.
(b) Block conversion of angiotensinogen to angiotensin I.

(c) Should not be used on patients with renal artery stenosis.
(d) May cause first-dose hypotension.
(e) Affect the metabolism of bradykinin.

41. Regarding shock:

(a) Results solely from acute blood loss.
(b) Is compensated for by Na^+ and water retention.
(c) Should always be treated with adrenaline.
(d) Only results in a fall in blood pressure with loss of >30% of blood volume.
(e) Peripheral vasoconstriction is a sign of hypovolaemic shock.

42. Compensatory mechanisms in heart failure include:

(a) Fluid retention through increased release of aldosterone.
(b) Tachycardia.
(c) Sympathetic activation.
(d) Venoconstriction.
(e) Arterial vasodilatation.

43. Angina:

(a) Is caused by ischaemic myocardium.
(b) Is never life-threatening.
(c) May be caused by atheromatous changes.
(d) Treatment involves increasing cardiac output.
(e) Can be treated with verapamil.

44. Atherosclerosis:

(a) Is only present in the elderly.
(b) Can affect veins as well as arteries.
(c) Predisposes to thrombosis.
(d) Is a complication of diabetes mellitus.
(e) Is a major cause of arterial stenosis.

45. Pathogenesis of atheroma is thought to:

(a) Involve platelets.
(b) Involve smooth muscle cells.
(c) Involve macrophages.
(d) Involve endothelial cells.
(e) Involve multiple cytokines.

46. In the treatment of hypertension:

(a) α-Adrenoceptor agonists are beneficial.
(b) Centrally acting drugs include methyldopa.
(c) Cyanide poisoning may result from administration of inorganic nitrates.
(d) Potassium channel agonists are reserved for refractory hypertension.
(e) Angiotensin II receptor antagonists are associated with dry cough.

47. Treatment of chronic heart failure:

(a) Aims to increase cardiac output.
(b) Should include digoxin.

(c) Can utilize β-blockers to reduce rate and force of contraction.
(d) May be treated using heart transplantation as a last resort.
(e) Works with the body's own compensatory mechanisms.

48. Myocardial infarction:

(a) Rapidly results in ST elevation.
(b) May lead to ventricular rupture and cardiac tamponade.
(c) Commonly results from platelet aggregation or thrombosis.
(d) May begin as a subendocardial infarction, which progresses to become transmural.
(e) Myocyte loss may continue even after reperfusion.

49. Medications which improve outcome following a myocardial infarction include:

(a) Aspirin.
(b) Angiotensin-converting enzyme (ACE) inhibitors.
(c) Calcium antagonists.
(d) Nitrates.
(e) β-Blockers.

50. In relation to lipid metabolism:

(a) Apolipoproteins act as docking proteins for lipoproteins.
(b) Oxidized LDL is chemotactic for macrophages.
(c) Type I hyperlipidaemia is treated by diet alone.
(d) Statins are a useful treatment for hypertryglyceridaemia (Type IV).
(e) Resins affect lipid metabolism in adipose tissue.

51. Regarding the pericardium:

(a) The pericardium normally contains 200 mL of fluid.
(b) Pericardial effusions may be serous, serosanguineous, or chylous.
(c) Cardiac tamponade is a medical emergency.
(d) Pericarditis is a recognized complication of rheumatoid arthritis.
(e) Serous effusions result from pericardial infection.

52. Syncope:

(a) May be caused by coughing.
(b) May be a sign of an intra-cardiac tumour.
(c) Associated with facial flushing suggests an arrhythmia.
(d) Is commonly caused by a vasovagal attack.
(e) May be caused by exercise in patients with mitral regurgitation.

53. Cardiomyopathy:

(a) The term cardiomyopathy implies a known aetiology.
(b) Cardiomyopathy is classified as restrictive, hypertrophic, or dilated.

(c) Restrictive cardiomyopathy is associated with an increase in ventricular mass.
(d) Excessive catecholamine levels may cause a dilated cardiomyopathy.
(e) Dilated cardiomyopathy may lead to heart failure, thromboembolism, and arrhythmia.

54. Endocarditis:

(a) Infective endocarditis is classified according to the infective organism.
(b) Commonly occurs after dental treatment.
(c) Is more common in drug addicts.
(d) May arise without an infection.
(e) Can result in peripheral emboli.

55. In the conducting system of the heart:

(a) The atrioventricular (AV) node is the normal pacemaker.
(b) The His bundle connects the sinoatrial (SA) node to the AV node.
(c) The right bundle has two branches.
(d) Conduction in the atria is faster than in the AV node.
(e) The sinoatrial node is found at the junction of the superior vena cava and right atrium.

56. Coarctation of the aorta:

(a) Is more common in men.
(b) Is associated with aortic dissection.
(c) Surgical correction should be avoided in childhood.
(d) May produce a weak left radial pulse.
(e) Is associated with bicuspid aortic valves.

57. In haemorrhagic shock there is:

(a) Decreased urinary output.
(b) Sweating.
(c) Thirst.
(d) Increased total peripheral resistance.
(e) Bradycardia.

58. Concerning hyperlipidaemia:

(a) Type II hyperlipidaemia typically raises cholesterol.
(b) Raised high-density lipoprotein (HDL) levels are a known risk factor for coronary heart disease.
(c) Hypercholesterolaemia is a common cause of pancreatitis.
(d) Diabetes mellitus is associated with some hyperlipidaemias.
(e) Pravastatin is an ion exchange resin that can be used to lower cholesterol levels in the blood.

59. Hypertension:

(a) Is defined by the World Health Organization as blood pressure above 140 mmHg systolic or 90 mmHg diastolic in any patient.
(b) Results exclusively from arteriolar smooth muscle contraction.

(c) Can be treated safely in the elderly with an angiotensin-converting enzyme (ACE) inhibitor.
(d) Control of blood pressure has no effect on cardiovascular morbidity.
(e) Many elderly patients also suffer from postural hypotension, so care must be taken in prescribing treatment.

60. In the treatment of arrhythmias:

(a) Amiodarone is used because it blocks Na^+ channels.
(b) β-Blockers can be used safely in asthmatics.
(c) Verapamil may make your skin turn blue in the sun.
(d) Digoxin can be used to treat atrial fibrillation.
(e) Atrial pacing can control atrial tachycardias.

61. In the management of myocardial infarction:

(a) Aspirin can reduce mortality.
(b) Streptokinase is used as the first-line treatment.
(c) Patients aged over 75 years will not benefit from thrombolysis therapy.
(d) A greater reduction in mortality can be achieved if treatment is started early.
(e) The use of recombinant tissue plasminogen activator (rt PA) lowers the reinfarction rate compared to the rate with streptokinase.

62. Heart failure:

(a) Occurs when the heart cannot pump enough blood to maintain adequate perfusion.
(b) Can be treated successfully with angiotensin-converting enzyme (ACE) inhibitors and thiazide diuretics.
(c) Milrinone is the first-line treatment.
(d) Is diagnosed by exercise echocardiography.
(e) Is characterized by bradycardia.

63. Coronary artery bypass grafting:

(a) Is more effective than medical therapy for relieving angina symptoms.
(b) Has a reduced risk of restenosis when compared with that of angioplasty.
(c) Commonly uses grafts made from artificial substances.
(d) Is routinely offered to all patients.
(e) Results in a reduced requirement for anti-anginal drugs when compared with angioplasty.

64. Acute left ventricular failure is accompanied by:

(a) An increase in pulmonary blood volume.
(b) Normal jugular venous pressure.
(c) Generalized vasodilatation.
(d) Ankle oedema.
(e) Raised arterial blood pressure.

65. Infective endocarditis can be associated with:

(a) Pain in the joints.
(b) Splinter haemorrhages.
(c) Patent ductus arteriosus.
(d) Heart murmurs.
(e) Intravenous drug abuse.

66. In congenital ventricular septal defects:

(a) Development of Eisenmenger's syndrome results in a left-to-right shunt.
(b) Small defects will usually close spontaneously.
(c) There is a pansystolic murmur.
(d) The murmur radiates to the neck.
(e) The defect usually involves the membranous part of the septum.

67. Risk factors for the development of ischaemic heart disease include:

(a) Elevated plasma low-density lipoprotein (LDL)-cholesterol concentration.
(b) Family history of non-insulin-dependent diabetes mellitus.
(c) Low factor VIII concentration in the blood.
(d) Obsessional personality.
(e) Smoking.

68. Concerning hypertension:

(a) Left ventricular hypertrophy improves with lowering of the blood pressure.
(b) Salt restriction helps lower blood pressure in some individuals.
(c) Is benign when hyaline changes occur in arteries.
(d) Is a major risk factor for atherosclerosis.
(e) Is caused by reduced compliance of large vessels.

69. In rheumatic fever:

(a) There is often a preceding group A β-haemolytic streptococcal infection.
(b) Skin rash may occur, particularly in children.
(c) There is a raised erythrocyte sedimentation rate.
(d) Small joint rather than large joint pain is typical.
(e) Large vegetations are present on the valves.

70. In hypertrophic obstructive cardiomyopathy:

(a) The pulse is slow rising.
(b) The systolic murmur characteristically decreases on squatting.
(c) Echocardiography is unhelpful.
(d) The right ventricle is never involved.
(e) 24-hour electrocardiographic monitoring may be useful to identify ventricular tachycardia.

71. Concerning cardiac tumours:

(a) Metastatic tumours are more common than primary tumours.
(b) Pulmonary embolism occurs in some patients with myxomas.
(c) Myxomas typically arise in the right atrium.
(d) Echocardiography is useful for identifying the location and shape of the tumour.

(e) They may mimic endocarditis with valve dysfunction and emboli.

72. Concerning chronic constrictive pericarditis:

(a) Paroxysmal nocturnal dyspnoea (PND) is a characteristic feature.
(b) Irradiation of the thorax is a recognized cause.
(c) Ascites and splenomegaly are typical features.
(d) Right and left ventricular end-diastolic pressures are equal.
(e) There is a prominent 'y' descent in the venous pressure caused by sudden brief filling of the right ventricle.

73. Coarctation of the aorta is associated with:

(a) Constriction just proximal to the left subclavian artery.
(b) A higher incidence of aortic stenosis.
(c) Marfan syndrome.
(d) A continuous murmur.
(e) Radiofemoral delay.

74. Risk factors for atherosclerosis include:

(a) Smoking.
(b) Raised high-density lipoprotein (HDL).
(c) Hypertension.
(d) Family history.
(e) Mediterranean-style diet.

75. Concerning dissecting aortic aneurysm:

(a) Aortic regurgitation is common.
(b) Pain often radiates to the back.
(c) It is essential to identify the point of re-entry so that surgery can be successful.
(d) Computerized tomography of the thorax is helpful in the diagnosis.
(e) May be caused by syphilis.

76. Concerning the vasculitides:

(a) Giant-cell arteritis often presents with headaches, temporal pain, and polymyalgia.
(b) Kawasaki disease usually occurs in children, and it can cause coronary aneurysms.
(c) Polyarteritis nodosa typically affects large arteries.
(d) Wegener's granulomatosis typically involves the lungs and kidneys.
(e) Thromboangiitis obliterans usually affects non-smokers.

77. Concerning haemangiomas:

(a) They more commonly affect children.
(b) Granuloma pyogenicum is a type of capillary haemangioma that occurs in pregnant women.
(c) They may present as strawberry naevi on the face of infants.
(d) Capillary haemangiomas are only found in the skin.
(e) They are benign tumours of blood vessels.

78. In deep-vein thrombosis:

(a) Most patients have ankle oedema.
(b) Pulmonary embolism can result in pyrexia.
(c) Doppler ultrasonography can be useful.
(d) Malignancy should be suspected if no obvious predisposing factor can be found.
(e) Lifelong treatment with anticoagulants should be given.

79. The following statements about β-blockers are correct:

(a) β-Blockers reduce blood pressure by vasodilatation.
(b) β-Blockers are used alone to treat hypertension caused by a phaeochromocytoma.
(c) β-Blockers reduce angina by dilating the coronary arteries.
(d) β-Blockers may be useful in the treatment of heart failure.
(e) β-Blockers are not very effective in the treatment of arrhythmias.

80. Electromechanical dissociation (EMD):

(a) Results in no activity on the electrocardiogram.
(b) Responds to defibrillation with DC cardioversion.
(c) Has a worse prognosis than ventricular fibrillation.
(d) Can be caused by cardiac rupture after a myocardial infarction.
(e) May respond to intravenous adrenaline.

Chapter 6—Common Presentations of Cardiovascular Disease

81. Cardiovascular presenting complaints may include:

(a) Syncope.
(b) Visual impairment.
(c) Nausea and vomiting.
(d) Shortness of breath at night.
(e) Neurological deficits.

82. Causes of central chest pain include:

(a) Dissecting aortic aneurysm.
(b) Pulmonary embolism.
(c) Pneumothorax.
(d) Oesophagitis.
(e) Pericarditis.

Chapter 7—History and Examination

83. The following pulse types are associated with these diseases:

(a) Pulsus alternans—left ventricular disease.
(b) Slow rising pulse—aortic stenosis.
(c) Collapsing pulse—hypotension.
(d) Pulsus paradoxus—cardiac tamponade.
(e) Pulsus bisferiens—pulmonary hypertension.

84. Classic abnormalities of the jugular venous pulse include:

(a) Absent 'a' waves in atrial fibrillation.
(b) Giant 'a' waves in tricuspid regurgitation.
(c) Large 'v' waves in pulmonary regurgitation.
(d) A slow 'y' descent in tricuspid stenosis.
(e) A raised jugular venous pressure on inspiration (Kussmaul's sign) with pericardial tamponade.

85. Correct findings on auscultation include:

(a) The first heart sound immediately follows the carotid pulse upstroke.
(b) Expiration causes physiological splitting of the second heart sound.
(c) A loud opening snap in diastole suggests mitral valve disease.
(d) The fourth heart sound, if present, coincides with atrial systole.
(e) A mid-diastolic click indicates mitral valve prolapse.

86. An ejection systolic murmur:

(a) Indicates aortic regurgitation.
(b) If found in the aortic area usually radiates to the neck.
(c) May be caused by an atrial septal defect.
(d) Is frequently caused by pulmonary stenosis.
(e) May be associated with an ejection click.

87. In inspiration:

(a) The murmur of a ventricular septal defect gets louder.
(b) Reverse splitting of the second heart sound occurs in pulmonary hypertension.
(c) Blood pressure falls with constrictive pericarditis.
(d) The heart rate is unaffected in the young.
(e) Pulmonary venous flow increases.

88. The following may be normal clinical findings in the elderly:

(a) A third heart sound.
(b) Dyspnoea on exercise.
(c) A diastolic murmur.
(d) Venous ulcers.
(e) Syncope.

89. Signs of cardiovascular disease include:

(a) Finger clubbing.
(b) Splinter haemorrhages.
(c) Peripheral ulcers.
(d) Palpable apex beat.
(e) Sinus arrhythmia.

90. The following heart sounds have these inferences:

(a) Splitting of the second heart sound on inspiration—left bundle branch block.
(b) Pansystolic murmur—mitral regurgitation.
(c) Ejection systolic—pulmonary stenosis.

(d) Mid-diastolic murmur—tricuspid stenosis.
(e) Continuous murmur—aortic stenosis and regurgitation.

91. When performing auscultation:

(a) The diaphragm is best suited to high pitched sounds.
(b) The pulmonary area is in the second intercostal space, left sternal edge.
(c) The tricuspid area is in the fifth intercostal space, left side.
(d) An abnormality heard in the aortic area should be checked for in the carotid artery.
(e) An abnormality heard in the mitral area should be checked for in the axilla.

Chapter 8—Investigations and Imaging

92. With regard to the ECG:

(a) Leads I–III are unipolar.
(b) Only 9 electrodes are used to generate signals for 12 leads.
(c) The appearance of the QRS complex varies because the electrical changes have amplitude and direction.
(d) Rhythm disturbance is best assessed by looking at lead III.
(e) The T wave is usually in the opposite direction to the R wave.

93. On an ECG:

(a) The anterior chest lead over the interventricular septum has equal R and S waves.
(b) The limb lead which is closest to the cardiac axis shows equal R and S waves.
(c) Einthoven's triangle can be used to find the cardiac axis.
(d) An R or S wave with a split and broadened peak is indicative of bundle branch block.
(e) An area of infarction may be located using an ECG.

94. Effective imaging techniques for specific disease include:

(a) Plain chest radiograph—pulmonary embolism.
(b) Computerized tomography—aortic aneurysm.
(c) Magnetic resonance imaging—myocardial hypertrophy.
(d) Doppler ultrasonography—peripheral vascular disease.
(e) Echocardiography—heart valve function.

95. Concerning electrical conductivity in the heart:

(a) The only way that the spread of excitation can move from the atria to the ventricles is through the atrioventricular node.
(b) There is a delay of 0.2 s between the impulse in the atrioventricular node and depolarization of the apex.

(c) The apex depolarizes last.
(d) The Purkinje system originates in the sinoatrial node.
(e) If there is a block in the wave of depolarization, no contraction occurs for an indefinite period.

96. Chest pain is likely to be caused by angina if:

(a) The onset is coordinated with exercise.
(b) Glyceryl trinitrate relieves the pain within 5 minutes.
(c) The pain radiates to the neck.
(d) The pain lasts for hours after rest.
(e) An exercise electrocardiogram shows ST elevation.

97. In the posteroanterior chest radiograph, the heart shadow:

(a) Will show left atrial enlargement.
(b) Is increased in right ventricular hypertrophy.
(c) Will show enlargement in hypertension.
(d) Is normally about 50% of the transthoracic diameter.
(e) Becomes enlarged in aortic stenosis.

98. In the electrocardiogram:

(a) Hypokalaemia produces flattened T waves.
(b) Right ventricular hypertrophy produces right axis deviation.

(c) Pathological Q waves are the first sign of infarction.
(d) A QT interval of 0.5 s is normal.
(e) Type II atrioventricular block shows lengthening of the PR interval.

99. Concerning cardiac enzymes:

(a) An increase in creatine kinase always indicates a myocardial infarction.
(b) Aspartate aminotransferase (AST) is also raised in liver disease.
(c) Electrocardiographic testing is not required if cardiac enzymes are raised.
(d) Lactate dehydrogenase reaches a peak within 24 hours.
(e) Troponin T tests are not as specific as the tests for cardiac enzymes.

100. Echocardiography:

(a) Involves the use of ultrasound waves to map the heart.
(b) Is not very good for looking at the movement of the heart and valves.
(c) Cannot be used for the diagnosis of dilated cardiomyopathy.
(d) Shows blood and fluid as a bright white colour.
(e) Can use the Doppler shift to look at blood flow through valves.

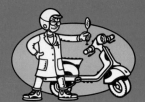

Short-answer Questions

1. Briefly describe the mechanisms by which noradrenaline increases intracellular Ca^{2+} concentration in vascular smooth muscle cells.

2. Blood flows through a straight vessel of radius (r) 0.1 cm and length 1.0 cm at a rate of 0.03 mL/min. At the input end the pressure, P_a, is 90 mmHg and at the outflow end, P_v, is 10 mmHg.

   (a) What will be the new flow if r increases to 0.2 cm with everything else constant?

   (b) What will be the new flow if the viscosity of the blood increases by 50% with everything else held constant at the original values?

   (c) What factors contribute to the viscosity of blood?

   (d) What will be the new flow if P_a falls to 50 mmHg with everything else constant at the original values?

3. (a) Explain what is meant by the term autoregulation?

   (b) Give an example of a vascular bed that shows good autoregulation.

   (c) What is the physiological importance of autoregulation in the tissue you have chosen?

4. Describe the carotid sinus baroreceptor reflex.

5. Outline the physiological mechanism by which blood pressure, volume, and composition are restored after haemorrhage.

6. What parasympathetic functions will be lost if the vagus nerves are bilaterally sectioned in the neck?

7. (a) What is meant by the term vasoactive metabolite?

   (b) Give two examples of vasoactive metabolites.

   (c) Give an example of a situation in which they are important.

8. (a) What event in the cardiac cycle is associated with the first heart sound?

   (b) What event in the cardiac cycle is associated with the second heart sound?

   (c) What is a cardiac murmur?

   (d) Give an example of a pathological condition that would give rise to a systolic murmur.

9. (a) What is meant by the term stroke volume?

   (b) Give the average value of end-diastolic volume of the left ventricle in a normal adult.

   (c) Give the average value of end-systolic volume of the left ventricle in a normal adult.

   (d) Give the average value of stroke volume of the left ventricle in a normal adult.

   (e) What factors determine the stroke volume?

   (f) What equations link:
   - Stroke volume to cardiac output.
   - Stroke volume to stroke work.

10. Draw a labelled diagram of a ventricular function curve (Starling curve), and show how this might be altered during sympathetic stimulation.

11. Describe the effects of adrenaline on the heart and blood vessels, and state which receptors are involved in the responses you describe.

12. (a) Along which routes can water and solutes cross the capillary endothelium?

    (b) What determines which route a molecule will take?

13. Outline the mechanism of action of the angiotensin-converting enzyme (ACE) inhibitors in the treatment of congestive heart failure.

14. A badly injured person has no overt loss of blood. If he is bleeding internally, what symptoms and signs of haemorrhage might be present?

15. (a) Explain how β-adrenoceptor antagonists (β-blockers) act on the cardiovascular system to relieve the symptoms of angina of effort.

    (b) Why are β-blockers not used to treat vasospastic angina (Prinzmetal's angina)?

16. Draw a labelled diagram of the cardiac cycle, including left ventricular and aortic pressures and the ECG.

17. (a) Outline the site and function of the ductus arteriosus in the fetus.

    (b) What causes it to close shortly after birth?

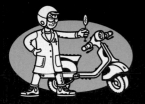

1. (a) True—The cardiovascular system is responsible for transporting many metabolites in plasma, including glucose and lipids.
   (b) True—Many hormones are soluble factors carried in the blood.
   (c) True—Local regulation of blood flow plays a key role in inflammation; immune cells and cytokines are carried in blood and lymph.
   (d) True—Temperature regulation is achieved by regulation of the circulation of the skin.
   (e) True—The cardiovascular system is responsible for an erection.

2. (a) True—The nodal artery supplies the AV node, branching off the right coronary artery.
   (b) False—The valves of the heart are avascular, receiving any metabolites from diffusion from the lumen.
   (c) False—Conduction through the AV node is relatively slow.
   (d) True—Adrenaline acts on β_2-receptors in the coronary arteries producing vasodilatation to increase myocardial perfusion.
   (e) True—Atrial natriuretic peptide forms part of the physiological regulation of blood volume; overstretch of the atria results from fluid overload.

3. (a) True—The resting membrane potential of contractile myocytes is –90 mV, predominantly through the concentration gradient of K^+ ions.
   (b) False—The developed tension in myocytes is proportional to cytoplasmic Ca^{2+} concentration, and so positive inotropes raise Ca^{2+} levels.
   (c) False—Intercalated disks form the structural junctions between myocytes while the gap junctions allow rapid electrical conduction.
   (d) True—Nodal, Purkinje fibre, and work cells are all examples of specialized myocytes.
   (e) True—The membrane potential of pacemaker cells declines partly through the leakage of Na^+ ions to threshold, when Ca^{2+} channels open.

4. (a) True—The oesophagus, aorta, and left main bronchus all lie behind (posterior to) the heart.
   (b) False—The diaphragmatic surface is formed mainly by the left ventricle.
   (c) True—The right ventricle forms most of the inferior border of the anterior surface.
   (d) True—The heart is enclosed by a double layer of serous pericardium.

   (e) False—The fossa ovalis is in the interatrial wall, not the atrioventricular wall.

5. (a) False—The aortic valve is tricuspid.
   (b) True—The AV node is connected to the ventricles via the bundle of His. In abnormal hearts, there may be additional pathways.
   (c) False—It is the left atrium that receives blood from the four openings of the pulmonary veins.
   (d) True—The papillary muscles ensure that the atrioventricular valves do not open when the ventricle contracts, preventing regurgitation.
   (e) True—All venous drainage of the heart passes through the coronary sinus into the right atrium.

6. (a) True—The resting membrane potential is maintained through the K^+ gradient, with Na^+ movement initiating depolarization.
   (b) True—Contractile myocytes are most permeable to K^+ ions.
   (c) False—The upstroke in nodal cells is relatively slow, and is dependent on an influx of Ca^{2+} ions.
   (d) False—The Nernst equation predicts the membrane potential resulting from an ionic concentration gradient.
   (e) False—In work myocytes, the upstroke is mediated by movement of Na^+ ions.

7. (a) True—Raised cytosolic Ca^{2+} triggers contraction.
   (b) True—An increased heart rate reduces the time for removal of cytoplasmic Ca^{2+} leading to raised levels of Ca^{2+} and, therefore, increased force.
   (c) True—Tension, or force of contraction, is proportional to cytoplasmic Ca^{2+} levels.
   (d) True—Changes that produce a higher resting Ca^{2+} level will lead to an increased force of contraction (see above).
   (e) False—Chronotropes affect the heart rate, not the strength of contraction.

8. (a) False—Development of the heart begins in week 3 of gestation.
   (b) False—The septum spurium is purely transient, while the septum primum and septum secundum separate the atria.
   (c) True—The truncus arteriosus undergoes a spiral process of septation to split the aorta and pulmonary trunk before rotating and separating.
   (d) True—The superior part of the inter-ventricular septum is a membranous extension of the fibrous skeleton of the heart.

(e) True—The single pulmonary vein becomes 4 through intussussception incorporating the first two branch points into the atrial wall.

9. (a) False—The epicardium is serous, not fibrous.
   (b) True—The innermost lining of the myocardium consists of vascular endothelium.
   (c) False—The myocardium contains Purkinje fibre cells as well as other cell types.
   (d) False—Myocardial muscle differs from skeletal muscle in several respects, including the branching structure and differing myofibril components.
   (e) True—Contraction of the myocardium must be coordinated to develop maximum tension. Islands of unresponsive myocardium may initiate arrhythmias.

10. (a) True—The action potential in the ventricles (the QT interval) lasts 0.3 s.
    (b) False—The opening of sodium channels give rise to the rapid upstroke.
    (c) True—The atrioventricular node can function as a pacemaker, but is normally suppressed by more frequent signals from the sinoatrial node.
    (d) False—Purkinje fibres are the fastest conducting cells in the conduction pathway. The slowest conduction occurs in the AV node.
    (e) True—Excitation and contraction are intimately linked; once intracellular ionic concentrations return to normal contraction ceases.

11. (a) False—Both ventricles are in series, and so eject equal volumes of blood. Muscle mass is greater in the left ventricle due to higher ejection pressures.
    (b) True—The mitral valve separates the left atrium and the left ventricle. As ventricular pressure falls during diastole the valve opens.
    (c) False—The first heart sound occurs at the beginning of isovolumetric contraction, when the atrioventricular valves close.
    (d) True—Isovolumetric contraction occurs at the start of systole as pressure increases to match the resistance to outflow.
    (e) False—Venous pressure is sufficient for some ventricular filling.

12. (a) False—The P wave is caused by atrial depolarization. The QRS complex is caused by ventricular excitation.
    (b) False—The PQ interval represents the time taken for the signal to cross the AV node. It is, therefore, not affected by atrial hypertrophy.
    (c) True—The QT interval corresponds to the ventricular action potential.
    (d) False—The first heart sound coincides with ventricular contraction (the QRS complex), the time the atrioventricular valves close.

(e) True—The peak of the R wave corresponds with the depolarization of the apex.

13. (a) True—CVP affects CO via venous return, while contractility and TPR will affect CO by altering outflow.
    (b) True—An increased end-diastolic pressure indicates greater filling of the ventricles, and hence greater volume, and vice versa.
    (c) False—The vagus nerve provides parasympathetic innervation, which reduces CO. Blocking vagal activity will increase CO.
    (d) True—Contractility is defined as the force of contraction for a given fibre length. An increased contractility therefore shifts Starling's curve to the left.
    (e) False—Exercise can increase the cardiac output to around 35 L/min in a normal subject (about a 7-fold increase).

14. (a) False—The force of contraction is directly proportional to the initial length of the muscle fibre.
    (b) False—Starling's law was first described in studies on isolated heart–lung preparations but is also valid physiologically.
    (c) True—The EDV determines the initial fibre length. This determines the force of contraction and hence the stroke volume.
    (d) False—Factors that reduce cardiac filling will reduce EDV and hence reduce the force of contraction.
    (e) False—Starling's law reflects the intrinsic properties of the cardiac myocytes, and does not depend on innervation.

15. (a) False—Cardiac output is the product of stroke volume and heart rate.
    (b) True—Contractility is affected by factors such as sympathetic stimulation.
    (c) True—End-diastolic volume and end-diastolic pressure are closely related because the relaxed ventricle stretches in response to increased pressure.
    (d) False—The Starling curve has a peak, but the downslope is caused by architectural distortion of the heart. Individual myocytes cannot be overstretched, unlike skeletal muscle.
    (e) True—This relation is the physiological equivalent of Ohm's law (i.e. resistance = pressure divided by flow).

16. (a) True—The intracellular receptor for EDRF is a guanyl cyclase.
    (b) True—Adrenaline binds to cell surface receptors, which activate adenylase cyclase.

(c) True—The transmitter used in sympathetic neuromuscular junctions is noradrenaline.

(d) True—Hypoxia causes hyperpolarization which reduces the number of open Ca^{2+} channels and hence reduces contraction.

(e) False—Smooth muscle is able to maintain tension for only 0.3% of the energy requirement of skeletal muscle.

17. (a) False—Hydrostatic pressure in the capillaries is highest at the arterial end.

(b) True—The effusion at the arterial end is greater than the reabsorption at the venous end, producing a net efflux.

(c) False—Metabolites move by diffusion and not with the fluid movements.

(d) True—Loss of plasma proteins reduces the oncotic pressure within plasma leading to a greater loss of fluid to the tissues.

(e) True—Lipid soluble molecules diffuse through EC in addition to the movement of soluble metabolites through fenestrations.

18. (a) True—Pulmonary resistance falls rapidly to allow greater volumes of blood to flow.

(b) False—During fetal development atrial pressures are equal, but the left atria develops a higher pressure after birth.

(c) True—Prostaglandins maintain the patency of the ductus venosus during gestation.

(d) True—The ductus venosus closes in response to the higher levels of oxygen in the blood from the aorta.

(e) True—The increased left atrial pressure seals the septum primum over the foramen ovale.

19. (a) True—Resistance varies inversely with the fourth power of the radius.

(b) True—Capillaries have the greatest total cross-sectional area of all vessel types.

(c) True—Blood pressure is the cardiac output multiplied by the total peripheral resistance.

(d) False—Vascular resistance is predicted by Poiseuille's law which describes the resistance to fluid flow.

(e) False—Vascular resistance is proportional to the length of the vessel.

20. (a) False—The vasculature consists of vessels designed for conductance, resistance, capacitance, and exchange.

(b) True—Arteries contain more smooth muscle than veins.

(c) False—The major resistance vessels are the arterioles and smaller arteries.

(d) False—Nutrients are also provided to larger vessels by the vasa vasorum in the adventitia.

(e) True—Metabolite supply and waste removal is the primary role of the cardiovascular system.

21. (a) True—Endothelium has a key role in regulating thrombosis and preventing clotting.

(b) False—The endothelium is responsible for local signals through cytokines and other molecules.

(c) True—Sympathetic release of adrenaline and noradrenaline generally cause vasoconstriction.

(d) False—Nitric oxide has a key role in maintaining the patency of vessels and regulating flow through smooth muscle relaxation and vasodilatation.

(e) True—Excitation triggers an increase in cytosolic Ca^{2+}, which causes contraction.

22. (a) True—Flow varies with the pressure difference and the resistance.

(b) False—Poiseuille's law determines resistance, such that flow is proportional to the radius to the fourth power.

(c) False—Similarly, flow is inversely proportional to the length (resistance is proportional to length).

(d) True—Increasing the viscosity increases the resistance and hence decreases the flow.

(e) True—Flow is defined as the volume of blood flowing per unit time, and is, therefore, dependent on the velocity.

23. (a) False—Veins contain about 60% of total blood volume. The capillaries only hold the blood involved in direct exchange.

(b) True—Red blood cells are forced to deform as they pass through the smallest capillaries to maximize gaseous exchange.

(c) True—Capillary sphincters control capillary blood flow, but do not contribute to resistance.

(d) True—Capillary walls also allow diffusion of water soluble molecules.

(e) False—Capillary walls are incapable of vasoconstriction. The arterioles are the resistance vessels.

24. (a) True—Extracellular or interstitial fluid is drained via the lymphatics.

(b) False—Lymph returns to the circulation through the subclavian vein.

(c) True—Lymphatic drainage ensures that antigens from the interstitial fluid are screened in lymph nodes.

(d) False—Lymph carries fats absorbed from the gut to the central circulation.

(e) False—Both brain and eye are unique in having their own systems for drainage.

25. (a) True—The renal arteries branch directly off the aorta in the abdomen.

(b) False—The internal iliac branches off the common iliac (which the aorta becomes).

(c) False—The right brachial artery is a branch off the right brachiocephalic trunk.

(d) False—The left colic artery is a branch of the inferior mesenteric artery.

(e) True—The inferior mesenteric branches off the abdominal aorta to supply the hindgut.

26. (a) True—The nodes receive direct innervation from both the vagus (parasympathetic) and sympathetic nervous systems.

(b) True—The myocardium receives direct sympathetic innervation.

(c) False—β_1-receptors are found in myocardium, while β_2-receptors predominate in peripheral vessels and in the bronchi.

(d) False—Cholinergic fibres innervate the SA and AV nodes, but not the ventricular muscle directly.

(e) True—Sympathetic activity can be blocked by vagal activity.

27. (a) False—Hyperpolarization mediates smooth muscle relaxation in response to hypoxia.

(b) True—Autoregulation is the process whereby vessel calibre automatically adapts to changes in perfusion pressure.

(c) False—Hyperaemia may be pathological, but is also physiological, e.g. in exercising muscle.

(d) False—There are sympathetic afferents which mediate vasodilatation in skeletal muscle.

(e) True—There are no parasympathetic vasoconstrictor nerves.

28. (a) False—Renin is released from the juxtaglomerular cells in the kidney.

(b) True—First discovered in extracts of brain tissue, brain natriuretic peptide is released from the ventricles in response to stretch.

(c) True—Vasopressin, otherwise known as anti-diuretic hormone, is released in response to an increased osmolarity.

(d) False—Angiotensin I is converted to angiotensin II by endothelial cells in the lung. Angiotensin II leads to vasoconstriction.

(e) True—Aldosterone acts on the renal tubules of the kidney to promote Na^+ and water retention.

29. (a) True—It may be reset by autonomic activity in, e.g. exercise, and also responds to flow and metabolic demand.

(b) True—Increased pressure leads to a greater tension in the vessel wall in order to increase resistance and regulate flow.

(c) False—Autoregulation acts to maintain constant flow at varying pressure, but is sensitive to metabolic demand.

(d) False—Myogenic autoregulation is achieved by the smooth muscle of the arterial walls and does not rely on innervation.

(e) False—The hyperpolarization and smooth muscle relaxation induced by hypoxia is a form of autoregulation.

30. (a) False—The responses to a fall in blood pressure act to maintain the blood flow to critical organs (e.g. brain) by vasodilatation.

(b) True—Vessels supplying skeletal muscle and other peripheral organs will vasoconstrict.

(c) True—Venoconstriction occurs by sympathetic activation to increase venous return and maintain cardiac output.

(d) False—Chemoreceptors in the aortic and carotid bodies will respond to a reduced blood pressure by stimulating ventilation.

(e) True—The baroreceptor response to reduced blood pressure includes increased sympathetic activation which increases cardiac contractility.

31. (a) True—As core temperature rises, blood flow to the skin rises to promote heat loss.

(b) True—Blood flow through the coronary arteries increases with increasing cardiac load.

(c) False—The volume of blood present in the pulmonary circulation at any one time is relatively small.

(d) True—There is little change in the metabolic demands on the cerebral circulation.

(e) True—The kidneys receive additional blood flow over and above their oxygen requirement due to their specialized role.

32. (a) False—During exercise, sympathetic activation anticipates the onset of exercise.

(b) False—The exercise pressor response stimulates cardiac output in response to exercise.

(c) True—Receptors for metabolites in skeletal muscle partly underlie the exercise pressor response.

(d) True—Peripheral vessels initially contract to maintain blood pressure but dilate as core temperature rises.

(e) False—Cardiac output may increase up to 7-fold, but this is achieved by increased heart rate with only a small increase in stroke volume.

33. (a) True—Training thickens the ventricular wall to meet the greater demands placed on the heart.

(b) True—Additional vessels develop within the myocardium to meet the greater metabolic demand.

(c) False—Cardiovascular training raises levels of myoglobin in skeletal muscle, but has no effect on haemoglobin levels.

(d) True—Skeletal muscle undergoes a similar improvement in vascularity.

(e) False—Athletes cannot raise their maximum heart rate through training, but may increase their cardiac output and muscle efficiency.

34. (a) True—Orthostasis is the term used to describe the changes that happen on rising from the supine position.

(b) True—Cardiac output falls as blood pools in the legs. The baroreceptors detect the resulting fall in blood pressure.

(c) True—On standing, gravity sets up an additional pressure gradient through the cardiovascular system.

(d) False—Sympathetically mediated vasoconstriction is a key component in maintaining blood pressure.

(e) True—Syncope may result if cerebral perfusion is not maintained.

35. (a) True—Fatigue and breathlessness are direct effects of the inability of the heart to maintain cardiac output.

(b) True—Breathlessness may be exacerbated by pulmonary oedema.

(c) True—Pulmonary oedema may also give rise to a nocturnal cough.

(d) True—Venous congestion from right-sided heart failure may cause liver enlargement.

(e) True—Pulmonary congestion from left-sided heart failure may lead to haemoptysis.

36. (a) False—This is a non-specific finding, and may arise from supraventricular or ventricular tachycardia.

(b) False—Carotid sinus massage may slow a tachycardia but does not differentiate supraventricular from ventricular causes.

(c) True—A variable intensity of the first heart sound is indicative of superventricular tachycardia; the others are less specific cardiac changes.

(d) False—Cardiac failure can arise from a range of non- cardiac causes.

(e) False—This is a non-specific finding with tachycardia, but does not indicate the origin.

37. (a) False—Supraventricular arrhythmias originate in the sinoatrial node of the atrial myocardium.

(b) False—Heart rates are considered normal between 60 and 100 beats per minute, although athletes may have a lower resting pulse.

(c) True—Sinus arrhythmia, a change in heart rate with respiration, is normal in the young.

(d) True—Wolf–Parkinson–White syndrome is caused by an extra conduction pathway and frequently causes tachycardia or atrial fibrillation.

(e) True—There is delayed conduction between the atria and the ventricles leading to an increased PR interval.

38. (a) True—The ventricles respond irregularly to the storm of signals passing down from the atria.

(b) True—Atrial fibrillation is a common finding in the elderly.

(c) True—Implanted pacemakers may be required to control chronic, intermittent episodes.

(d) True—Atrial fibrillation is one of many complications of thyrotoxicosis.

(e) False—Atrial fibrillation may lead to serious complications (e.g. stroke through thromboembolism) but is rarely directly fatal itself.

39. (a) True—Amiodarone may cause a fibrosing alveolitis.

(b) True—Many drugs may cause liver damage in individual patients.

(c) False—Constipation is a side effect of verapamil.

(d) False—Exacerbation of asthma is a risk accompanying the use of β-blockers.

(e) True—Amiodarone contains iodine and is a recognized cause of thyroid disorders.

40. (a) True—Angiotensin-converting enzyme is most highly expressed on pulmonary vascular endothelium.

(b) False—Angiotensin-converting enzyme converts angiotensin I to angiotensin II.

(c) True—By blocking the physiological response to impaired renal perfusion ACE inhibitors may precipitate renal failure.

(d) True—ACE inhibitors should be prescribed with care.

(e) True—Angiotensin-converting enzyme is also responsible for the breakdown of bradykinin, a pro-inflammatory cytokine.

41. (a) False—Shock can result from haemorrhage, dehydration, anaphylaxis, and many other causes.

(b) True—The body compensates for fluid loss by retention of water and Na^+.

(c) False—Cardiogenic shock from chronic heart failure should not be treated with adrenaline.

(d) True—Physiological compensatory mechanisms initially defend blood pressure.

(e) True—Sympathetic activation to maintain cardiac output and blood pressure results in peripheral vasoconstriction.

42. (a) True—Reduced renal perfusion leads to increased renin and aldosterone secretion.

(b) True—In response to failing perfusion the body tries to compensate by increasing heart rate.

(c) True—Heart failure is accompanied by compensatory sympathetic activation, which attempts to preserve blood pressure and cardiac output.

(d) True—Venoconstriction reduces the volume of blood stored in the veinous circulation, increasing venous return.

(e) False—There is widespread arterial vasoconstriction to maintain blood pressure.

43. (a) True—Overexertion of the heart beyond the available blood supply creates ischaemia.

(b) False—Unstable angina is a serious condition, as 15% of cases progress to a myocardial infarction. Classical angina of effort is not life-threatening.

(c) True—Atheromatous changes are the most common cause of stenosis.

(d) False—Treatment for angina aims to reduce the work of the heart and increase the coronary blood flow.

(e) True—Verapamil blocks Ca^{2+} channels, producing vasodilatation and reducing arterial resistance.

44. (a) False—Early atheromatous changes will already be present in most people of university age.

(b) False—It only affects the arteries, as the venous system operates under low pressure with significantly reduced shear stress.

(c) True—Injured or denuded endothelium is a risk factor for thrombosis.

(d) True—Diabetes mellitus is a strong risk factor for atherosclerosis.

(e) True—Atheromatous changes are the leading cause of arterial stenosis.

45. (a) True—Platelet derived growth factor (PDGF) released by adherent platelets is a potent smooth muscle mitogen.

(b) True—Smooth muscle cell migration from the media into the intima is a key pathogenic step.

(c) True—Macrophages are recruited into the atherosclerotic lesion where they oxidize LDL and secrete growth factors.

(d) True—Atherosclerotic changes are likely to be initiated by endothelial injury.

(e) True—Many cytokines are involved in the recruitment and multiplication of cells in atherosclerotic lesions.

46. (a) False—α-Adrenoceptors mediate constriction in the vasculature, and so should be blocked.

(b) True—Methyldopa is a centrally acting antihypertensive reserved for use in pregnancy.

(c) True—Cyanide poisoning is a serious risk with use of sodium nitroprusside.

(d) True—Potassium channel agonists hyperpolarize smooth muscle cells, producing vasodilatation. Side effects limit their use.

(e) False—Angiotensin II receptor antagonists can be tried if ACE inhibitors produce an intolerable cough by elevating levels of bradykinin.

47. (a) False—Treatment of chronic heart failure aims to reduce the work done by the heart, which may reduce cardiac output.

(b) False—Digoxin is commonly used in chronic heart failure to increase contractility but does not prolong life.

(c) True—β-blockers inhibit sympathetic activity, reducing cardiac load.

(d) True—Heart transplantation is a treatment of last resort due to the highly invasive surgery and long-term immunosuppression required.

(e) False—Therapy aims to manage the body's compensatory mechanisms to reduce cardiac work and prevent further pathological changes.

48. (a) True—ST elevation occurs within hours of myocardial infarction.

(b) True—The affected region of the heart may rupture up to several days after a myocardial infarction causing cardiac tamponade.

(c) True—Platelet aggregation or thrombosis from an atherosclerotic lesion are frequent causes of myocardial infarction.

(d) True—Incomplete vessel occlusion may produce a sub-endocardial infarct that progresses with complete occlusion.

(e) True—Reperfusion injury occurs when blood flow is re-established, and so there may be further loss of myocytes after thrombolysis.

49. (a) True—Antiplatelet effects of aspirin are beneficial.

(b) True—ACE inhibitors have been shown to prolong life.

(c) False—Calcium antagonists are beneficial for angina.

(d) False—Nitrates are used in the management of angina.

(e) True—β-Blockers are beneficial following myocardial infarction.

50. (a) True—Lipoproteins are composed of lipids and apolipoproteins. The apolipoproteins have several roles.

(b) True—Oxidized LDL is likely to play a significant role in attracting macrophages into atherosclerotic lesions.

(c) True—Type I hyperlipidaemia is characterized by raised triglyceride levels alone, and is treated by dietary control.

(d) False—Statins inhibit HMG CoA reductase, which is involved in endogenous synthesis of cholesterol. They have no effect on triglyceride levels.

(e) False—Fibrates act on adipose tissue to reduce activity of lipoprotein lipase.

51. (a) False—A normal pericardium may contain 50 mL of fluid.

(b) True—Effusions may arise from blood, interstitial fluid, or lymph.

(c) True—Cardiac tamponade prevents adequate cardiac filling and must be drained.

(d) True—Pericarditis occurs in 30% of patients with severe, chronic rheumatoid arthritis.

(e) False—Serous effusions result from heart failure or hypoproteinaemia.

52. (a) True—Cough is a recognized respiratory cause of syncope.

(b) True—A tumour that exerts pressure on or invades the aorta may produce syncope.

(c) False—Syncope associated with arrhythmia (Stokes–Adams attacks) are associated with pallor.

(d) True—The most common cause of fainting is a vaso-vagal attack, triggered by pain or other emotional stimulus.

(e) False—Valvular changes are not associated with syncope on exertion.

53. (a) False—The term cardiomyopathy is generally used for conditions where the pathogenesis is unknown.

(b) True—Cardiomyopathy is functionally classified.

(c) False—Restrictive cardiomyopathy is associated with stiffening of a normal size ventricular wall.

(d) True—Chronic, excessive levels of catecholamines may lead to dilated cardiomyopathy.

(e) True—Excessive dilatation leads to poor cardiac function, which may lead to heart failure, mural thrombi, or arrhythmias.

54. (a) True—Current schemes classify the disease according to the infective organism.

(b) True—Oral or pharyngeal pathogens may enter the bloodstream after dental treatment.

(c) True—Intravenous drug abusers risk introducing pathogenic organisms into their blood.

(d) True—Non-bacterial thrombotic endocarditis may arise through clotting disorders.

(e) True—Sequelae of endocarditis include valve incompetence, embolic disease, and renal complications.

55. (a) False—The normal pacemaker of the heart is the SA node.

(b) False—There is no specialized conduction pathway between the SA and AV node. The bundle of His carries signals from the AV node.

(c) False—The bundle of His splits to form the right and left bundle branches, which then connect to Purkinje fibres.

(d) True—Conduction in the AV node is slow to allow time for complete contraction of the atria.

(e) True—The SA node lies in the posterior wall of the right atrium.

56. (a) True—The male:female ratio is 2:1.

(b) True—Aortic dissection is a recognized complication.

(c) False—Surgery to correct coarctation of the aorta should be performed as soon as possible.

(d) True—Coarctation often impairs blood flow to the left arm and lower limbs, but not the right arm.

(e) True—Bicuspid aortic valves are found in about 50% of cases.

57. (a) True—Urine output is minimized to reduce fluid loss.

(b) True—Sympathetic activation leads to sweating and peripheral vasoconstriction.

(c) True—Increased thirst is part of the physiological response to fluid loss.

(d) True—Total peripheral resistance is increased to maintain blood pressure and maintain essential organ perfusion.

(e) False—Tachycardia is a common sign in haemorrhagic shock.

58. (a) True—Raised cholesterol is a major feature of type II hyperlipidaemia.

(b) False—High levels of HDL are protective against atherosclerosis and CHD.

(c) False—High levels of triglycerides may lead to pancreatitis.

(d) True—Diabetes mellitus has many effects on metabolism.

(e) False—Statins act on HMG CoA reductase to reduce endogenous cholesterol synthesis.

59. (a) False—The definition of hypertension also depends on age; higher limits are set for blood pressure in the elderly.

(b) False—Causes of hypertension are diverse and multifactorial.

(c) True—ACE inhibitors are widely used in the treatment of hypertension.

(d) False—Reduction of blood pressure, even within the range defined as normal, will reduce mortality.

(e) True—Normal physiological defence of blood pressure weakens with age.

60. (a) False—Amiodarone acts on K⁺ channels.

(b) False—β-Blockers, even if cardioselective, still exert some effects on β_2-receptors in the bronchi, worsening asthma.

(c) False—Skin discolouration and photosensitivity are side effects of amiodarone.

(d) True—Digoxin has a central effect via the vagus causing partial atrioventricular block.

(e) True—Atrial pacing may control atrial tachycardias through overdrive suppression from the pacemaker.

61. (a) True—The anti-platelet effects of aspirin have been demonstrated to be beneficial.

(b) True—Streptokinase is the current first-line thrombolytic, but not should be used repeatedly for the same patient.

(c) False—All patients may benefit from thrombolysis.

(d) True—Irreversible ischaemic injury and reperfusion injury may both be minimized by rapid intervention.

(e) True—Controlled trials have demonstrated a reduced reinfarction rate for rtPA versus streptokinase.

62. (a) True—The failure of the heart to maintain adequate tissue perfusion is one of the key steps in the development of chronic heart failure.

(b) True—ACE inhibitors unload the heart while thiazide diuretics counter the fluid retention of chronic heart failure.

(c) False—Treatment is aimed principally at reducing the load on the heart, and so milrinone is reserved for later use.

(d) False—Heart failure is characterized by ventricular dilatation, which may be detected on normal echocardiography.

(e) False—Compensatory mechanisms frequently include tachycardia.

63. (a) True—CABG may cure the patient's angina, while medical treatment is aimed at symptomatic relief.

(b) True—Restenosis may occur after both angioplasty and CABG, but at a lower incidence following CABG.

(c) False—Grafts are taken from the patient's own vasculature.

(d) False—Bypass grafting is usually only offered to patients with severe or refractory angina.

(e) False—Patients often still require anti-angina medications after angioplasty or CABG.

64. (a) True—Left ventricular failure increases pulmonary pressure. The distensibility of the pulmonary circulation leads to increased volume.

(b) True—In chronic heart failure, fluid retention will increase the central venous pressure.

(c) False—Generalized vasoconstriction occurs to maintain blood pressure.

(d) False—Chronic failure will lead to fluid retention and oedema.

(e) False—In acute left ventricular failure, the failure of the heart as a pump leads to a fall in blood pressure.

65. (a) True—Infective endocarditis is associated with a systemic inflammatory reaction, producing flu-like symptoms.

(b) True—Splinter haemorrhages are a common sign of infective endocarditis.

(c) True—Individuals with a patent ductus arteriosus are at increased risk.

(d) True—Damage to the heart valves often causes murmurs.

(e) True—Intravenous drug abuse increase the chances of introducing bacteria into the circulation.

66. (a) False—Eisenmenger's syndrome occurs when the normal left-to-right shunt is reversed, with blood going from right to left causing cyanosis.

(b) True—Small defects can be asymptomatic and close spontaneously.

(c) True—Movement of blood occurs throughout systole with symptomatic VSD.

(d) False—The murmur does not usually radiate.

(e) True—VSD most commonly arises from failure of fusion of the membranous and muscular ventricular septa.

67. (a) True—Elevated LDL is associated with increased risk of IHD through increased atherosclerotic plaque formation.

(b) True—Diabetes is a potent risk factor for IHD.

(c) False—Loss of Factor VIII leads to haemophillia.

(d) False—An obsessional personality is a recognized risk factor for hypertension, but not directly for ischaemic heart disease.

(e) True—Smoking is a recognized risk factor for IHD through endothelial injury.

68. (a) True—Left ventricular hypertrophy most commonly arises through systemic hypertension. Unloading the heart will reverse the hypertophy.

(b) True—Reduced salt intake is beneficial for hypertensive individuals.

(c) True—Hyaline changes in arteries are associated with benign hypertension.

(d) True—Hypertension increases the stress placed on vascular endothelium, predisposing to atherosclerotic changes.

(e) True—Reduced compliance prevents normal vessel expansion.

69. (a) True—Streptococcal septicaemia is a common precursor to rheumatic fever.

(b) True—Erythema marginatum (a macular rash with erythematous edge) occurs more frequently in children.

(c) True—Rheumatic fever is an autoimmune, systemic inflammatory disease. The ESR is frequently raised.

(d) False—The joint pain in rheumatic fever typically affects the large joints.

(e) False—Rheumatic fever is associated with small, bead-like vegetations on the heart valves.

70. (a) False—The pulse is jerky.

(b) True—The murmur arises from obstruction to cardiac outflow and is classically reduced on squatting.

(c) False—HOCM may be diagnosed by echocardiography to assess heart size.

(d) False—It may be assymetrical but frequently affects both left and right ventricles.

(e) True—Intermittent episodes of tachycardia may best be detected using 24-hour monitoring.

71. (a) True—Primary cardiac tumours are extremely rare.

(b) True—Myxomatous masses may fragment to produce emboli.

(c) False—75% of cardiac myxomas arise in the left atrium.

(d) True—Echocardiography is a useful and non-invasive investigation to visualize the heart.

(e) True—Systemic responses to cancer may lead to non-bacterial thrombotic endocarditis.

72. (a) False—PND is a general feature of heart failure, and is therefore not characteristic of constrictive pericarditis.

(b) True—Fibrosis of the pericardium producing constrictive pericarditis is a recognised complication of thoracic radiotherapy.

(c) True—Constrictive pericarditis leads to systemic venous congestion, which may lead to abdominal complications.

(d) True—Limited space for ventricular expansion means that the EDP in both ventricles must be equal.

(e) True—Venous congestion raises the central venous pressure, which falls rapidly during ventricular diastole.

73. (a) False—The stenosis in coarctation is found distal to the left subclavian artery.

(b) True—Coarctation of the aorta may occur alongside other congenital abnormalities, including aortic stenosis.

(c) False—Marfan syndrome is associated with aortic aneurysms and valve defects, but not coarctation.

(d) False—Coarctation of the aorta usually causes an ejection systolic murmur.

(e) True—The aortic constriction weakens and delays the strength of the femoral pulse.

74. (a) True—Smoking causes vascular endothelial injury, promoting atherosclerosis.

(b) False—HDL is beneficial in reducing the incidence of atherosclerosis.

(c) True—Chronic hypertension imposes greater stress on the vascular endothelium, predisposing to atherosclerosis.

(d) True—Family history is a strong predictor of risk.

(e) False—A Mediterranean-style diet rich in olive oil and fresh produce is protective.

75. (a) True—Extension of the tear towards the valves may disrupt their function.

(b) True—Chest pain with radiation to the back suggests aortic aneurysm.

(c) False—Surgery is the definitive treatment for a dissecting aortic aneurysm, but there may or may not be a re-entry point.

(d) True—Computerized tomography using contrast medium is the optimal imaging technique.

(e) True—Aortic aneurysms are a recognized complication of syphilis.

76. (a) True—Giant-cell (temporal) arteritis may also lead to blindness.

(b) True—20% of patients will have coronary arteritis with aneurysms.

(c) False—Polyarteritis nodosa more commonly affects the small to medium size arteries.

(d) True—Necrotizing vasculitis of the lungs and glomerulonephritis forms part of the classical presentation.

(e) False—Thromboangiitis obliterans usually affects young men who smoke.

77. (a) True—Haemangiomas are common, especially in children.

(b) True—Ulcerated haemangiomas are known as granuloma pyogenicum and affect 5% of pregnant women.

(c) True—Juvenile capillary haemangiomas appear at birth, but usually disappear by age of 5 years.

(d) False—Capillary haemangiomas may also occur in mucosal membranes.

(e) True—Haemangiomas make up approximately 7% of all benign tumours.

78. (a) False—Most patients with a deep vein thrombosis are asymptomatic.

(b) True—Fever is a recognized symptom of pulmonary embolism.

183

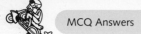

(c) True—Doppler ultrasonography is useful to identify blocked blood vessels.

(d) True—Primary or secondary pulmonary tumours may give rise to the symptoms of pulmonary embolism.

(e) False—Lifelong treatment with anticoagulants is only indicated for patients with persistent hypercoagulable states or repeated episodes.

79. (a) False—β-Blockers act to reduce cardiac output by blocking sympathetic drive, reducing the metabolic load on the heart.

(b) False—Phaeochromocytomas should be treated surgically, with α-antagonists used first.

(c) False—β-Blockers help to manage angina by reducing cardiac work.

(d) True—Unloading the heart is beneficial in heart failure.

(e) False—Conduction is also slowed, making β-blockers beneficial in arrhythmia.

80. (a) False—EMD occurs when there is normal electrical activity without corresponding output.

(b) False—Electrical activity is normal, the underlying problem is not an arrhythmia.

(c) True—EMD is a serious sign and is rapidly fatal without reversal of the precipitating factors.

(d) True—Serious cardiac rupture will lead to cardiac tamponade, and if untreated, EMD.

(e) True—Adrenaline may increase contractility to support what little cardiac output remains.

81. (a) True—Syncope may result from inadequate cerebral perfusion.

(b) True—Visual impairment may also result from limited cerebral perfusion.

(c) True—Nausea and vomiting may indicate malignant hypertension.

(d) True—Paroxysmal nocturnal dyspnoea is an indication of heart failure.

(e) True—Neurological deficits may indicate a stroke or transient ischaemic attack.

82. (a) True—The pain of a dissecting aortic aneurysm is usually sharp and radiates towards the back.

(b) True—Pulmonary emboli typically give rise to a localized, sharp chest pain.

(c) False—The pain associated with a pneumothorax is usually felt laterally and not centrally.

(d) True—Oesophagitis commonly gives rise to a burning retrosternal pain.

(e) True—The pain of pericarditis is usually associated with breathing or movement.

83. (a) True—Alternating strong and weak pulses indicate severe left ventricular disease.

(b) True—Aortic constriction reduces maximum flow through the aortic valve.

(c) False—A collapsing pulse is characteristic of aortic regurgitation.

(d) True—A pulse that weakens or disappears on inspiration may be caused by asthma, cardiac tamponade, or pericarditis.

(e) False—A combination of slow rising and collapsing pulse indicates both aortic stenosis and regurgitation.

84. (a) True—The 'a' wave is caused by atrial contraction. Without coordinated activity this pressure wave does not occur.

(b) False—Giant 'a' waves are an indication of tricuspid stenosis, not regurgitation.

(c) False—Large 'v' waves are characteristic of tricuspid regurgitation, or constrictive pericarditis.

(d) True—The 'y' descent corresponds with the opening of the tricuspid valve and is slow with a stenosed valve.

(e) True—JVP is raised on inspiration with cardiac tamponade and constrictive pericarditis.

85. (a) False—The first heart sound occurs before ejection, and so will be heard before the pressure wave is palpable in the carotid artery.

(b) False—Physiological splitting of the second heart sound is observed on inspiration.

(c) True—The mid-diastolic click indicates the opening of an abnormal mitral or tricuspid valve.

(d) True—The fourth heart sound results from reduced ventricular compliance producing abnormal filling.

(e) False—The sound of a mitral valve prolapse is heard in mid-systole, not diastole.

86. (a) False—Aortic regurgitation produces a diastolic murmur.

(b) True—Murmurs identified in the aortic area indicate abnormalities of aortic flow, and will also be audible over the carotid arteries.

(c) True—Ejection systolic murmurs best heard at the left sternal edge suggest an atrial septal defect.

(d) False—Pulmonary stenosis is uncommon.

(e) True—Abnormal valve sounds may be associated with an opening click or snap.

87. (a) False—Pulmonary stenosis gives rise to a murmur that is louder on inspiration.

(b) False—P_2 is loud with pulmonary hypertension, but no splitting occurs.

(c) True—Constrictive pericarditis limits cardiac expansion, limiting stroke volume and cardiac output. Symptoms of heart failure result.

(d) False—Sinus arrhythmia is a normal finding in the young.

(e) False—Reduced thoracic pressures on inspiration increase the volume of blood in the pulmonary circulation but reduce the venous flow to the left atrium.

88. (a) False—A third heart sound may be normal in young adults or in pregnancy, but not in the elderly.

(b) True—Poor exercise tolerance is a normal finding in the elderly, without suggesting serious pathology.

(c) False—Diastolic murmurs are never innocent.

(d) False—Venous ulceration is a common complication of varicose veins and impaired peripheral circulation.

(e) False—Syncope without obvious cause should be investigated.

89. (a) True—Finger clubbing is a non-specific indication of disease, but may occur with infective endocarditis or congenital heard disease.

(b) True—Splinter haemorrhages are classically seen in infective endocarditis.

(c) True—Peripheral ulcers are a sign of poor peripheral circulation and may indicate deep-vein thrombosis or peripheral arterial disease.

(d) False—A palpable apex beat is normal, and only indicates disease when it is found outside the normal area or is accompanied by heaves or thrills.

(e) False—Sinus arrhythmia is the natural variation in heart rate between inspiration and expiration.

90. (a) False—Splitting of the second heart sound on inspiration is a normal finding.

(b) True—The murmur of mitral regurgitation is pansystolic.

(c) True—Ejection systolic murmurs may indicate pulmonary or aortic stenosis.

(d) True—Mitral stenosis or tricuspid stenosis give rise to mid-diastolic murmurs.

(e) True—Continuous murmurs throughout systole and diastole suggests aortic stenosis and regurgitation.

91. (a) True—The bell is best suited for low pitched sounds.

(b) True—This is where you would listen for abnormal sounds from the right ventricle and pulmonary valves.

(c) False—The fifth intercostal space on the left sternal edge is the mitral area.

(d) True—Abnormalities heard in the aortic area may be audible over the carotid artery.

(e) True—Abnormalities heard in the mitral area may

radiate to the axilla.

92. (a) False—Leads I–III are bipolar.

(b) True—6 unipolar and 3 bipolar electrodes are used to generate the 12 'leads'.

(c) True—The QRS complex changes in character between the different leads.

(d) False—Rhythm disturbances are best assessed by looking at lead II, which is closest to the normal cardiac axis.

(e) False—The T and R waves are in the same direction due to the delayed repolarization of the interventricular septum relative to the apex.

93. (a) True—The wave of depolarization progresses down the septum, passes the electrode and progresses through the external ventricular walls.

(b) False—A limb lead which shows equal R and S waves is at right angles to the cardiac axis.

(c) True—Einthoven's triangle is drawn using the relative sizes of the QRS wave in the bipolar leads I to III and shows the direction of the cardiac axis.

(d) True—Blockade of either bundle branch slows conduction through the affected ventricle.

(e) True—Abnormal Q waves are indicative of an infarcted region in the outer ventricular wall directly beneath an anterior chest lead.

94. (a) False—Plain chest X-rays will rarely show signs of a pulmonary embolism. Ventilation–perfusion studies or pulmonary angiography are required.

(b) True—Computerized tomography using contrast medium allows precise measurement of the size of the aneurysm.

(c) True—MRI with contrast media allows accurate determination of the size of the heart and the chamber volumes.

(d) True—Doppler ultrasonography allows direct observation and quantitation of blood flow through peripheral vessels.

(e) True—Echocardiography is a highly effective technique for monitoring heart valve function.

95. (a) True—The normal heart has only one specialized pathway for atrioventricular (AV) conduction.

(b) False—Ventricular conduction is fast, taking only 80 ms for a signal to reach the apex from the AV node.

(c) False—The apex depolarizes before the myocardium of the external ventricular walls.

(d) False—The signal travels down the interventricular septum, reaches the apex and continues via Purkinje fibres through the external ventricular wall.

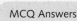

(e) False—A block in the conduction path can be overcome by 'escape' rhythms.

96. (a) True—The additional work required of the heart during exercise predisposes to ischaemia.
(b) True—Glyceryl trinitrate is a potent and rapid acting vasodilator, which will relieve angina through action on the coronary arteries.
(c) True—Pain radiating to the neck, jaw or shoulder are all classic signs of a cardiac origin.
(d) False—Classical angina is relieved by rest; this is a cardinal sign.
(e) False—Ischaemia results in ST depression on an exercise electrocardiogram, although ST elevation may be seen following a myocardial infarction.

97. (a) True—The left atrium forms the superior and left supero-lateral border of the heart shadow.
(b) False—In the PA radiograph the heart shadow is predominantly cast by the left ventricle.
(c) False—Hypertension will only show changes when left ventricular heart failure develops due to hypertrophy from chronic overload.
(d) True—This is a good general guide to the size of the heart.
(e) True—Left ventricular hypertrophy from the obstruction to outflow will be visible on the PA radiograph.

98. (a) True—Hypokalaemia is a correctable cause of altered T waves.
(b) True—Increased myocardial muscle mass causes deflection of the cardiac axis towards the affected side.

(c) False—Pathological Q waves are slow to develop, appearing within days.
(d) False—A normal QT interval is 0.4 s.
(e) False—A constant PR interval is seen with Mobitz type II heart block.

99. (a) False—Creatine kinase may also be released from skeletal muscle and brain.
(b) True—AST is also found in liver, lung, kidney, and red blood cells.
(c) False—An ECG may confirm the nature of the injury and may help to localize the lesion.
(d) False—Lactate dehydrogenase usually peaks after 2–3 days.
(e) False—Troponin T is unique to cardiac cells, and so is a more specific test for myocardial injury.

100. (a) True—Echocardiography uses ultrasound to visualize the heart and its movements.
(b) False—Echocardiography is the method of choice to investigate the movements of the heart and the heart valves.
(c) False—Echocardiography is also used to assess cardiac size.
(d) False—Blood appears black, unless Doppler shift is measured, when colour is used to depict blood flow on an echocardiogram.
(e) True—Doppler ultrasonography uses the changes in the reflection of sound waves from moving objects.

SAQ Answers

1. Varicosities on sympathetic nerves release noradrenaline (NA), which diffuses to α-adrenergic receptors on smooth muscle fibres. The G-protein coupled adrenergic receptor activates the cell via the cAMP second messenger pathway. Activation of the cell increases the intracellular calcium concentration by the following mechanisms:
   - Rapid release of Ca^{2+} from sarcoplasmic reticulum.
   - Receptor-gated Ca^{2+} channels in the sarcolemma.
   - Voltage-gated channels in the sarcolemma.
   - Caveolae, which are invaginations in the sarcolemma analogous to T tubules and are important in the smooth muscle uptake of Ca^{2+}.

2. (a) According to Poiseuille's law: flow = (pressure difference) $\pi r^4/\eta L$. If r doubles then r^4 increases by 16 times (2^4). This implies that flow also increases by 16 times. Thus, flow = 0.48 mL/min.

   (b) η increases by 50% = η multiplied by 3/2. As η is a denominator for the flow equation then flow must change by a factor of 2/3 (i.e. Flow = original flow $\times$ 2/3). Thus, flow = 0.02 mL/min.

   (c) Factors contributing to the viscosity of blood are:
   - Haematocrit.
   - Plasma proteins—globulins and albumin.
   - Temperature.
   - Radius—viscosity is greater in arterioles where the marginal layer (where the cells are close to the walls) makes up a greater proportion of the lumen. Also, viscosity is less in capillaries where single file flow occurs.
   - Velocity—if flow rate is low cell agglutination occurs.

   (d) Pressure difference = $P_a - P_v$ = 90–10 originally = 80 mmHg originally. New pressure difference = 50–10 = 40 mmHg now. This means that the pressure difference has halved and this implies that flow will be halved. Thus flow = 0.015 mL/min.

3. (a) Autoregulation is the process by which the flow of blood remains constant even though the blood pressure may change. This only occurs over a limited range of pressures. The process is independent of nervous control and is due to the myogenic response and a vasodilator effect.

   (b) Cerebral (or renal, intestinal, coronary, skeletal muscle).

   (c) For small changes in pressure the perfusion of the brain will be maintained. Also autoregulation has a protective role, preventing capillary damage and oedema formation.

4. The baroreflex buffers short-term fluctuations in blood pressure. An increase in pressure causes increased stretch of the baroreceptors. This stretch increases the rate of firing of these receptors. This information is conveyed to the medulla. It results in an increase in parasympathetic drive and decreased sympathetic drive. This produces bradycardia, decreased contractility, peripheral vasodilatation, and reduced blood volumes—caused by aldosterone, angiotensin II and antidiuretic hormone (ADH) suppression. In this way the blood pressure is reduced back to normal.

   A fall in blood pressure has the opposite effect.

5. The physiological responses to haemorrhage are shown in Figs 5.1–5.3.

6. Cardiac functions lost:
   - Vagal inhibition of the sinoatrial (SA) node, producing bradycardia.
   - Negative inotropic effect on atrial contraction (decreases atrial contractility).

   Vascular functions lost (generally a vasodilator effect) are:
   - Salivary gland vasodilatation (secretions will dry up with loss of vagus supply).
   - Pancreatic vasodilatation (drying up of secretions).
   - Intestinal vasodilatation (drying up of secretions).
   - Coronary artery vasodilatation (minor effect).
   - Cerebral artery vasodilatation.

   Other functions lost include:
   - Cough reflex.
   - Speech (via recurrent laryngeals). Often cut accidentally.

   Genital erectile tissue vasodilatation is not lost because it has a sacral parasympathetic innervation.

7. (a) A vasoactive metabolite is a product of metabolism in a tissue that produces an action on the vascular smooth muscle of the supplying vessel. This action is usually relaxation of the smooth muscle producing vasodilatation.

   (b) Lactate, adenosine, carbon dioxide, phosphate, K^+.

   (c) In exercising muscle, the rise in the level of local metabolites produces vasodilatation. This increases the blood supply to the muscle and facilitates an increased metabolic rate enabling the muscle to contract.

8. (a) Closure of the mitral and tricuspid valves.

   (b) Closure of the aortic and pulmonary valves.

   (c) Turbulent blood flow at or around an abnormal valve or valve ring.

   (d) Aortic stenosis produces an ejection systolic murmur. Mitral regurgitation produces a pansystolic murmur.

9. (a) Stroke volume is the volume of blood ejected from the ventricle in each ventricular contraction.

   (b) 120 mL.

   (c) 50 mL.

   (d) 70 mL.

   (e) Stroke volume can be influenced by:
   - Contractility—an increase in contractility increases stroke volume.
   - Initial myocardial stretch—increased stretch (i.e. increased EDV) will increase stroke volume according to Starling's law.
   - Arterial pressure—raised arterial pressure (an increase in afterload) opposes ejection, therefore decreasing stroke volume.

   (f) Equations are:
   - Cardiac output (CO) = stroke volume (SV) × heart rate.
   - Stroke work (SW) = SV × arterial pressure.

10. See Fig. 2.51.

11. Physiological concentration of adrenaline is 0.1–0.5 nmol/L. When secreted, concentration can rise to 5 nmol/L. Adrenaline causes:
   - Increased heart rate and contractility: β1-receptors.
   - Vasoconstriction in all tissues at high concentrations: α_1-receptors.
   - Vasodilatation at physiological concentrations in skeletal muscle, myocardium and liver: β_2-receptors.

   Overall adrenaline secretion causes a decrease in total peripheral resistance and an increase in cardiac output. There is an increase in mean blood pressure.

12. (a) Routes by which water and solutes can cross the capillary endothelium are:
   - Transcellular—lipophilic molecules (e.g. O_2, CO_2).
   - Intercellular—small pores—small lipophobic molecules (e.g. water, ions).
   - Fenestrations—small lipophobic molecules (e.g. water).
   - Transendothelial-large pores—large molecules (e.g. proteins, lymphocytes).
   - Vesicular transport—large lipophobic molecules (e.g. proteins).

   (b) Factors determining the route molecules will take are:
   - Lipid solubility.
   - Molecular size.
   - Type and permeability of capillary.
   - Pressure gradient (especially for water).
   - Concentration gradient (for other solutes).

13. Angiotensinogen $\xrightarrow{\text{renin}}$ angiotensin $\xrightarrow{\text{ACE}}$ angiotensin II

   ACE inhibitors block the action of ACE. Therefore they prevent the formation of angiotensin II. Angiotensin II:
   - Stimulates secretion of aldosterone.
   - Vasoconstriction.
   - Increases cardiac contractility.

   In congestive heart failure preventing angiotensin II formation has the following beneficial actions:
   - Decreased secretion of aldosterone and, therefore, increased salt and water excretion.
   - Prevention of vaso and venoconstriction decreasing cardiac filling pressure and afterload.
   - Causes vasodilatation, improving cardiac output.

14. Symptoms and signs of haemorrhage are:
   - Feeling faint/light-headed/dizzy.
   - Altered level of consciousness.
   - Pale, cold, clammy skin.
   - Rapid, weak pulse.
   - Reduced pulse pressure.
   - Rapid, shallow breathing.
   - Impaired renal output.
   - Muscular weakness.
   - Confusion or reduced awareness.

15. (a) β-Blockers prevent the sympathetic stimulation of β-receptors of the heart. They have the following actions in angina:
   - Decrease heart rate and therefore prolong diastole and perfusion time for the myocardium.
   - Decrease oxygen demand of the myocardium by decreasing contractility and heart rate.

   (b) Vasospastic angina is caused by spasm of the coronary arteries and this is probably an α-adrenoreceptor-mediated action. β-blockers have no dilatory effect on coronary arteries and so have no effect in vasospastic angina.

16. See Fig. 2.38.

17. (a) The ductus arteriosus passes from the root of the left pulmonary artery to the inferior concave surface of the arch of the aorta. It serves to bypass the non-functioning lungs in the fetus so that blood is shunted straight into the systemic circulation from the right side of the heart.

   (b) The ductus arteriosus closes 1–8 days after birth. It is thought that as the pulmonary circulation fills, the drop in pressure in the pulmonary trunk causes blood to flow from the aorta into the pulmonary trunk through the ductus arteriosus. This blood is oxygenated and the increase in P_{O_2} causes the smooth muscle in the wall of the ductus to constrict. This obstructs flow in the ductus arteriosus. Eventually the intima of the ductus arteriosus thickens and complete obliteration results in the formation of the ligamentum arteriosum, which attaches the pulmonary trunk to the aorta.

18. (a) Inotropic is the term used for anything that changes the contractility and therefore the force of contraction of the heart (e.g. dobutamine is a positive inotropic agent as it increases contraction). Chronotropic is the term used for any

substance that alters the rate of contraction of the heart. Any agent that increases the heart rate is called a positive chronotropic agent and anything that slows the heart rate is a negative chronotropic agent.

(b) An example of a positive chronotropic agent is noradrenaline.

19. (a) Muscle blood flow is increased by:
- Metabolic vasodilatation due to vasoactive metabolites (e.g. adenosine, K^+, H^+).
- Capillary recruitment.
- Skeletal muscle pump, which increases venous return and, therefore, increases the pressure gradient between arterial and venous systems, driving more blood through the capillaries.
- There may also be a central alerting response, which has a sympathetic vasodilator action on muscle vasculature and also increases cardiac output.

(b) At lower temperatures paradoxical cold vasodilatation occurs in an attempt to minimize cell damage. When the skin temperature is between 10 and 15 degrees vasoconstriction and venoconstriction occur in the hand. There is an abundance of α_2-receptors in the skin vessels. When the temperature falls these receptors have an increased affinity for noradrenaline. Noradrenaline causes the vascular smooth muscle to constrict, leading to vasoconstriction and, therefore, decreased flow.

20. The baroreflex that is elicited on standing leads to vaso and venoconstriction, which counteracts the loss of blood from the thoracic compartment and the fall in cardiac output caused by standing. On continued standing, the skeletal muscle pump and the valves in the veins play the main role in aiding venous return. Contraction of extrinsic skeletal muscle compresses the vein, and this increases venous pressure. As there are valves in the veins preventing retrograde flow then blood can only move towards the heart. This method facilitates venous return to the thoracic compartment.

The respiratory pump may also play a small role in aiding venous return. The intrathoracic pressure falls during inspiration, and this has a suction effect on the venous blood, driving it into the great veins.

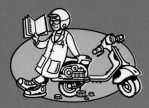

Index

Page numbers in *italics* refer to figures and tables.

A

A (anisotropic) band 17, *19*
abdomen
　arteries *35*
　auscultation 141
　examination 141–2
　palpation *142*
　percussion 141
　veins *36*
abdominal aortic aneurysms
　40, 85
accessory hemiazygos vein *34*
ACE *see* angiotensin-converting
　enzyme
acetylcholine 60
actin 18, 43–4, *45*
action potential 18, *20*, *21*
acute coronary syndromes 121
adenosine 95, *96*
adenosine triphosphate (ATP)
　18, *19*
adhesive pericarditis 102
adrenaline 61
　calcium (Ca^{2+}) channels 18
　control of blood flow 61, 65,
　　66
　therapeutic use 95
　see also catecholamines
adrenergic neuron blockers 78
adriamycin toxicity 101
adverse drug effects
　anaphylactic 90
　chemotherapy 110
　hypotension 123
　types A and B 79
African Kaposi's sarcoma 111
afterload 28, *29*
ageing
　baroreceptors 62
　blood pressure and 47, 62
　cerebral circulation 66
AIDS 112
alcohol intake 128
alcoholic cardiomyopathy 99,
　100

aldosterone 61–2, 68
alinidine 96
α-adrenoreceptors 57, 61
α$_2$-agonists, centrally acting 78
alpha-blockers 77–8
amiodarone 95, *96*
amlodipine 78
amyloidosis 100, 101
anaphylactic shock 73–4, 90
anaphylactoid reaction 74
ANCA *see* antineutrophil
　　cytoplasmic
　　autoantibodies
aneurysms 85–6
　aortic *see* aortic aneurysm
　berry 85, 86, 109
　Charcot–Bouchard 76
　congenital 86
　false 85
　left ventricle *156*
　mycotic 85
　true 85
anger *see* emotion
angina 87–8, 121
　drug treatment 87–8
　of effort (classic) 87, 88
　pain 121, *122*
　stable 87
　surgical treatment 114–15
　unstable 87
　vasospastic (Prinzmetal's) 87,
　　88
angioblastic cords 10, 34
angiography 150–1, 155, *157*,
　　158
angiomatosis, bacillary 111
angioplasty, balloon 114–15
angiosarcoma 111
angiotensin 61–2, 68
angiotensin II receptor
　　antagonists 77
angiotensin-converting enzyme
　　(ACE) 62
　inhibitors 76–7, 78–9, 92
angular artery *37*

angular vein *37*
anistreplase (APSAC) 90
ANP *see* atrial natriuretic
　　peptide
anterior cerebral artery *38*
anterior circumflex artery *39*
anterior communicating artery
　　38
anterior facial vein *37*
anterior inferior cerebellar artery
　　38
anterior interosseous artery *39*
anterior tibial artery *40*
anterior tibial vein *41*
antiarrhythmic drugs 94–5, *96*
　classification
　　Sicilian Gambit 95
　　spreadsheet approach *96*
　　Vaughan–Williams 94–5
antidiuretic hormone
　　(ADH/vasopressin) 61,
　　68
antihypertensive drugs 76–9
antineutrophil cytoplasmic
　　autoantibodies (ANCA)
　　102–3
aorta 3–4, 10, *35*, *42*
　coarctation 40, 75, 107, *108*
　development 34, 35, 40
　pressure 4
　thoracic *11*, *34*
aortic aneurysms
　abdominal *40*, 85
　dissecting 85–6, 121, 130,
　　159
　syphilitic (luetic) 85
　thoracic *159*
aortic arch 6, *7*
　baroreceptors 62
　development 34
　syndrome (Takayasu's
　　disease) 103
aortic body 64
aortic regurgitation 96, 97
aortic sinus 9